Private Residential Care: The Admission Process and Reactions of the Public Sector

JUDITH PHILLIPS

Social Work Development Unit
School of Economic and Social Studies
University of East Anglia

Avebury

Aldershot · Brookfield USA · Hong Kong · Singapore · Sydney

Published by
Avebury
Ashgate Publishing Limited
Gower House
Croft Road
Aldershot
Hants GU11 3HR
England

Ashgate Publishing Company
Old Post Road
Brookfield
Vermont O5036
USA

A CIP catalogue record for this book is available from the British Library and the US Library of Congress

ISBN 1 85628 188 4

Printed in Great Britain by
Athenaeum Press Ltd, Newcastle upon Tyne.

Contents

List of tables		vii
List of diagrams		x
Acknowledgements		xii
Foreword		xiii
CHAPTER 1:	LITERATURE REVIEW	1
CHAPTER 2:	METHODOLOGY	48
CHAPTER 3:	PROFILE OF PRIVATE RESIDENTIAL HOMES AND THEIR OWNERS	73
CHAPTER 4:	PROFILE OF RESIDENTS ENTERING PRIVATE RESIDENTIAL CARE	92
CHAPTER 5:	THE JOURNEY INTO RESIDENTIAL CARE	112
CHAPTER 6:	PRIVATE RESIDENTIAL CARE: PREFERENCE OR PRAGMATIC CHOICE?	145
CHAPTER 7:	KEY OPERATORS IN THE PROCESS OF ADMISSION: HOME OWNERS AND THEIR SELECTION PROCESS	176

CHAPTER 8: KEY OPERATORS IN THE PROCESS OF ADMISSION: RELATIVES AND PROFESSIONALS 191

CHAPTER 9: THE PROCESS OF ADMISSION INTO PRIVATE RESIDENTIAL CARE 227

POSTSCRIPT 239

Bibliography 245
Name index 260
Subject index 263

List of tables

1.1	Numbers of elderly people in Great Britain 1901-2021	2
1.2	The need for care in Great Britain 1971-2001	5
1.3	Public expenditure and expenditure on social welfare as percentage of gross national product 1900-1973	6
1.4	Expenditure on supplementary benefit payments for private home residents (England and Wales)	34
2.1	Sample areas for study	56
2.2	Number of homes covered in each area	57
2.3	Reason for non-response of resident	64
2.4	Reason for non-response of relatives	64
2.5	Composition of professionals named as 'Significant Other'	65
2.6	Summary of interview rates	66
3.1	Origin and former function of the thirty-nine private residential homes	75
3.2	Location of homes studied	76
3.3	Ownership/management of private residential homes	79
3.4	Segregated roles of husband and wife in private residential care management	80
3.5	Previous occupational background of private sector home owners	80
3.6	Age structure of home owners	81
3.7	Length of operation	82
3.8	Motivations in becoming a home owner	82

4.1	Age distribution in private and public sectors of care	93
4.2	Gender of residents entering private and local authority residential care	96
4.3	Marital status of residents	96
4.4	Gender and marital status of residents in private and local authority care	97
4.5	Social class of residents	98
4.6	Primary source of funding in the private sector	98
4.7	Residents' ownership of housing	99
4.8	Financial source and ownership of property of residents in the private sector	100
4.9	Social class and property ownership of residents	100
4.10	Physical condition: dependency of residents in residential care	102
4.11	Physical condition and gender of residents entering private residential care	103
4.12	Summary classification of dependency	105
4.13	Ratings of confusion: residents in private and local authority residential care	107
4.14	Marital status of women and their levels of confusion in the private sector	107
5.1	Type of residents' former housing	113
5.2	Geographical location of residents prior to admission	115
5.3	Composition of residents' former housing	116
5.4	Informal support at home	118
5.5	Services received prior to admission	119
5.6	Informal support to men at home	120
5.7	Background factors to admission into private and local authority residential homes	122
5.8	Specific factors leading directly to admission into private and local authority homes	123
5.9	Source of admission	137
5.10	The nature of admission	138
5.11	Source and nature of admission	139
6.1	Alternatives available to private and public sector residents	148
6.2	Options within residential care	148
6.3	Significant 'others' involved in the process of admission and options available to private sector residents	150
6.4	Source of admission and options available in the private sector	151
6.5	Why community care/living at home was not followed as an alternative to private residential care	152
6.6	Reasons for deciding between public and private residential care	159
6.7	Why this particular home?	167
6.8	Residents' satisfaction with services in private homes	169

6.9	Residents' happiness with life in private homes	169
6.10	Factors associated with happiness and satisfaction	170
7.1	Source of referrals	178
8.1	Significant 'others' in the process of admission	192
8.2	Age profile of carers	193
8.3	Whose decision to enter residential care?	196
8.4	Significant 'others' in admission to private homes and residents' source of admission	202
8.5	Circumstances under which social workers were involved in the private sector	204
8.6	Circumstances under which elderly people did not have a social worker involved in their private sector admission	205
8.7	Level of social work activity in the private residential care admission process	215

List of diagrams

1.1	Residential accommodation for persons aged 65 years and over in England (1976-1987)	33
2.1	Residential care for elderly people in Suffolk: local authority, private and voluntary sectors compared (1984)	52
2.2	County of Suffolk	54
2.3	Distribution and proportion of local authority and private registered beds in four chosen areas of Suffolk (1985)	55
4.1	Age and sex distribution in private and public sectors of care	94
4.2	Private and local authority homes compared by age and sector	95
4.3a	Dependency scale: physical condition	101
4.3b	Amalgamated dependency scores	102
5.1	The extent of overlap between private and public sectors	141
6.1	Residents' choice of public or private residential care	160
6.2	Professional views of private homes studied	171
7.1	Stages of admission into private residential care: home owners' perspective	179

7.2	Levels of physical and mental dependency of resident acceptable to private home owners	186
7.3	Amalgamated scores for accepted level of dependency	187
9.1	The percentages of residents who exercise a preference for private or public sector care	233

My sincere thanks and
gratitude to all the elderly
people and their families, whose
help and openness I could not have done
without. Thank you for making
the research enjoyable

Foreword

In 1979 changes in the supplementary benefit system allowed a wider range of elderly people, who otherwise would have remained at home or sought public sector residential care, to gain access to private residential care. As a result of such policy changes there was a phenomenal rise in the number of elderly people entering private residential homes. In the light of these developments, this book seeks to understand why and how elderly people entered private residential care. Interviews were conducted with elderly people, their carers, key professionals and home owners in an attempt to describe and explain the process of admission into residential care in the county of Suffolk.

Privatization has effected the provision of residential care for elderly people more than any other sphere of welfare. Between 1979 and 1984 the number of places provided in England by private homes increased by 93% (Wistow, 1987a). The meteoric rise in the number of residential homes for elderly people in the private sector was partly due to a response to the increasing number of frail elderly people unable to remain at home because of a decline in the number of available carers. The burgeoning number of private homes also followed a series of policy moves promoting a private sector of welfare; but whether such moves were intended to lead to an explosion in private care and were specifically designed to further the government's drive towards privatizing welfare is debateable.

Whatever the intention, the result of increasing private sector residential care contradicts the government's stated commitment to a policy of community care. The objective of keeping elderly people at home for as long as possible is undermined by placing resources in favour of enabling people to seek a private home rather than remain in the community. Such policy also undermines the public sector of welfare. In other words, at a time of financial restraint and local government ratecapping, state finance is pumped into an alternative private system. The government appears, therefore, to be actively shifting the balance of care from the public sector to the private sector operating under market principles.

It could be said that this shift is necessary in order to accommodate the increasing numbers of elderly people seeking a residential placement and it could also be argued that a decline in public sector places is a natural consequence of the consumer rejecting a provision of an inferior quality. The negative image of public sector residential care has permeated much of the writing on residential care from Townsend (1962) onwards. Institutional care, it is stated by its critics such as Townsend (1962) and Phillips et al (1988), promotes extreme forms of dependency, restricts choice and is encumbered by bureaucratic hurdles of various kinds, particularly in relation to admission. Alternatively, it is argued by economists like Seldon (1981) that through competition the private sector produces a better quality product: the elderly person entering this sector, therefore, would select the 'best' provision from a variety of homes on offer in the market and in this way 'cowboy' proprietors would go out of business.

There is, however, very little empirical evidence to support the argument that the private sector promotes greater choice or is a better quality product. Research to date shows that most elderly people view residential care, in any sector, as a last resort and would prefer to remain at home for as long as possible. Very few elderly people exercise a positive choice for residential care: an admission to care is often a response to circumstances such as increasing frailty or a breakdown in support networks which are often beyond the control of the elderly person.

Much of the evidence for and against admission to residential care relates to admission into the public sector. There is little qualitative research on the private sector to explain the process of admission. The phenomenal and alarming growth of private residential homes, their organisational framework and the response of the local authorities to such growth through regulation has been widely reported since 1980. Other literature concentrates on the few examples of exploitation and abuse of elderly people in private homes. However, there is a lack of description and explanation in the literature of the processes operating in admission to private residential care. The reasons why people go into private rather than public sector homes, the information concerning the persons with whom prospective residents discuss their options and how the choice between different private homes is made are missing pieces from the body of knowledge on this sector. In other words, there is no theoretical framework to explain the process of supply and demand operating in relation to the private sector.

This book attempts to redress the balance and looks at the extent to which similar people enter public and private care, under what circumstances they enter and the extent to which their separate journeys into the two sectors take them along similar lines.

In relation to the process of admission into public and private residential care, the book concludes that:

a) there were wide ranging similarities in the characteristics and

circumstances of people who entered both sectors. The differences emerged only in respect of mental state, social class and home ownership: private sector residents were less likely to be confused, tended to come from a wealthier social class and were previously home owners.
b) the differences between the two sectors emerged in respect of the support elderly people received in their process of admission. Relatives were the main source of guidance in the private sector process, whereas social workers were the main operators in the public sector. The presence of a relative and absence of a professional in the process of admission became a determining factor in the eventual decision to enter a private residential placement.

Relatives looked naturally at the private sector first, seeing themselves free in the process of admission to negotiate directly with the home owner. They saw no necessity to include social workers in their discussions because the latter were seen only as gatekeepers to scarce local authority resources and were not viewed as key professionals in the admission process to private homes.

These findings resulted from two hundred interviews with residents recently admitted to thirty nine private homes in Suffolk, together with one hundred and twenty local authority residents who also entered residential care within a period of one year. Alongside this consumer perspective, relatives and professionals who were identified as 'significant' others and the thirty nine home owners gave their views of the process of admission in respect of their influence and role. The presentation of this book is timely in relation to the future direction of services for elderly people. Local authorities with overall responsibility for the welfare of elderly people can no longer ignore the real challenge of private sector growth. They will have to include the private sector in their planning mechanism and decision making. Such a move will not only be a challenge to planners and managers but will pose certain difficulties at a practical level if social workers are to work within and alongside an alternative system of welfare. Social workers as public sector agents will need to look at their own role in working with elderly people, many of whom will seek a residential placement in the private sector and may not wish to involve a social work professional in that process.

The increasing role of relatives and redundancy of social workers in the private residential care process is interesting as the future of residential care increasingly becomes a private sector provision.

The rise of private sector provision in the overall context and development of welfare for elderly people is reviewed through the literature in the first chapter. Moving away from the literature-based research, Chapter Two describes the methodology employed in the empirical study.

Chapter Three looks at the supply side of the equation in the private care sector and gives the researcher's impression of the thirty nine private homes and describes the profile of home owners. The characteristics of their customers, the residents, are described in Chapter Four which highlights some of the main differences between residents in the public and private sectors. Chapters Five and Six focus on the journey into residential care. Chapter Five covers the circumstances leading to admission and Chapter Six the choice or preference expressed between public and private care and looks at alternatives open to elderly people.

The choice of home may not rest with the resident but with those people helping the elderly person in their search for a suitable home. The eventual outcome may also depend on the selection process of the home owner. Chapters Seven and Eight address these issues by describing the process of admission from a number of different 'viewing' points - particularly those of home owners, relatives and social workers.

Finally the relationship between all these interested parties is explored in relation to the development of welfare for elderly people in Chapter Nine which also draws together the major themes of the book.

1 Literature review

Although the topic of this book is specific to a relatively small part of the United Kingdom, and although it deals with a particular element in the admission of elderly people into private and public sector homes, the findings, and the discussion must be viewed within the context of political and historical traditions which have created the systems under analysis.

Accordingly, this chapter will attempt to put the process of admission into private residential care into a broader framework by reviewing relevant literature in three associated areas: first, it will discuss the place of elderly people in the UK and consider the question of responsibility for them and their welfare; second, having indicated the extent to which that responsibility is accepted by the state even to the extent of providing total care for the most dependent, it will explore the idea of residential care in the public sector; and third, it will highlight the emergence of a renewed emphasis on private sector provision since 1980 and consider both research evidence and political and economic arguments for and against it. In each main section, particular attention will be paid to the place of the social worker.

Responsibility for the welfare of elderly people

1. Demographic trends

An unique twentieth century phenomenon: an ageing population. Significant shifts in the demographic structure of the UK have taken place during this century, particularly in relation to the numbers of elderly people in the population. More elderly men can now expect to live up to 16 years on average in retirement (20 years for women) through improvements in environmental conditions and nutrition (Norton et al, 1986). Along with this decline in mortality, there has been a long-term downward trend in fertility, thus producing an unique twentieth century phenomenon: an ageing population.

Table 1.1 outlines the historical trends from 1901 and the predicted number of elderly people in Great Britain until 2021.

TABLE 1.1
NUMBERS OF ELDERLY PEOPLE IN GREAT BRITAIN: 1901 - 2021

	Age 65+		Age 75+		Age 85+	
	No.	%	No.	%	No.	%
Past trends						
1901	1734	4.7	507	1.4	57	0.15
1931	3316	7.4	920	2.1	108	0.24
1951	5332	10.9	1731	3.5	218	0.45
1971	7140	13.2	2536	4.7	462	0.86
1981	7985	15.0	3052	5.7	552	1.03
Current situation: 1983 - 1988						
1983	8246	15.1	3377	6.2	620	1.1
1986*	7739	-	3292	-	639	-
1988	8697	15.8	3736	6.8	757	1.4
Future trends: 1988 -2021						
1988	8697	15.8	3736	6.8	757	1.4
1991	8795	15.9	3844	6.9	757	1.4
2001	8656	15.3	4082	7.2	1047	1.9
2011	8911	15.7	4053	7.1	1187	2.1
2021	9956	17.2	4401	7.6	1230	2.1

No. = 000s.
% = percentage of total population of Great Britain
Source: Phillipson & Walker (1986, p.5). Population projections by the Government Actuary. Mid-1981 based principal projection 1981-2021 and OPCS Census data 1901-81. From *1986 the source is OPCS. Monthly digest of statistics June 1987.

In 1901 elderly people constituted about 5 per cent of the total population in Great Britain with fewer than 3 out of every 10 over 75 years of age. Although there was a steady increase in the first half of the century, from 1931 to 1981 the numbers of people aged 65 and over doubled and those over 75 quadrupled. This gradual increase in the numbers of 'old' elderly people is likely to continue and it has been estimated that the number of those aged 75 and over will increase by 18 per cent between now and the end of the century and those 85 and over by around 50 per cent (Norton et al, 1986 p.10). It is not this increase in numbers, however, that is interesting but the fact that the increase involves a heterogeneous group of people.

'Moral panic'. The size of the ageing population and marked growth of the very old population presented in the literature above have been exaggerated and used to keep alive the image of elderly people constituting a threat or burden to society. Sheldon's 1948 report of an inquiry in Wolverhampton captures such anxiety about numbers and led to the setting up of a Royal Commission on the Population in 1949 to look at the 'burden of dependency'. Sheldon stated:

> much anxious thought will be needed to arrive at a solution that shall be fair both to those who, having already served their generation, feel entitled to some measure of peace and happiness in their remaining years, and to those of the younger generation on whose shoulders this task has necessarily to be placed. (Sheldon 1948, p.1)

An historical overview also reveals that periods of demographic panic or fiscal crisis raise the political status of elderly people (McCoy, 1986). The 'burden of dependency' debate again reopened with the fiscal crisis in the 1970's with the projected trends in numbers seen as a 'drain on economic recovery'. Titmuss (1958), however, believed that the alarm was unjustified and that demographic changes were exaggerated. Any emphasis on current unprecedented growth is a mistake (Blaikie & MacNicol, 1986). However, alarming increases in the elderly population continue to be emphasised in much of the literature on old age and as a result 'moral panic' over projected numbers, has continued. One recent example was provided in 1983 when the Health Advisory service published a report warning of the 'rising tide' of elderly people suffering mental infirmity.

Phillipson & Walker, however, while acknowledging the trends, provide refreshment to the rather gloomy picture presented by demographic commentators. They make efforts to establish that elderly people are not a burden on the economy or society:

> The burden of dependency thesis has hindered an understanding of the true nature of dependency in old age. We are encouraged to believe that the social problem of dependency exists just because the numbers in a particular age group are increasing, by the simple but mistaken translation of demographic projections into social realities. (Phillipson & Walker 1986, p.11)

Despite such recognition the development of policy in residential and community care has been influenced by such literature emphasis on increasing numbers of dependent elderly to the extent that the focus has been on the implications of the increase rather than how best to meet the needs of elderly people.

Implications of an ageing population. It is not the size but the heterogeneity of the population over 60 that constitutes a social problem to policy makers and planners. No one model or stereotype of ageing described by the literature can fit such a population.

Although the majority of elderly people are fit, well and independent (Norton et al, 1986), one of the major consequences of old age is the prevalence of illness which increases with advancing years (Hunt, 1978; Shanas et al, 1968). Specific problems of limited mobility, incontinence and dementia affecting elderly people occur in significant proportions. Hunt (1978) found that 60 per cent of the over 75's reported themselves as suffering from long standing illness, disability or infirmity. Nearly 20 per cent of those aged over 85 were bedfast and 51 per cent were unable to bath themselves.

Allied to the demographic trends are other social trends which are significant for the understanding of the experience of old age and the arrangement for care in old age in this country. For example, the living status of elderly people, decreasing family size and economic consequences of old age.

There has always been a significant proportion of elderly people living alone (Wall, 1984) and although not intrinsically undesirable for this group of 40 per cent of the over 75's (1981 figs. OPCS), this situation does compound the problem of how their care needs will be met and by whom.

Although the family still provides the main source of care for elderly people (Tinker, 1981) there have been several changes in the composition of the family which have resulted in the reduction of the number of close relatives acting as care-givers. The share of the burden for those able to care has therefore increased.

Elderly people are often also viewed in much of the literature as an 'economic burden' in a capitalist society dominated by concepts of production, growth and market forces. Leonard (in Phillipson, 1982) argues that they are seen as non-productive and redundant in such a society. Large numbers of elderly people are dependent financially on the state through pensions and other benefits and are generally more likely to live on the margins of poverty, particularly if widowed (Anderson, 1974). In 1980/1 almost three-quarters of elderly people compared with a fifth of non-elderly lived in or on the margins of poverty (DHSS, 1983). A consequence of this is the need for increased public spending to cope with increasing numbers of relatively 'poor' people.

Rossiter and Wicks (1982, p.57) show that the overall expenditure on health and personal social services in 1978/79 was £300 per head for people aged 65-74, yet £805 per head for those over 75. Such expenditure for this latter group will need to continue rising as it grows rapidly in numbers.

The current cuts in the rate support grant and measures of rate-capping imposed on local government, however, have major implications for local authorities in terms of meeting the increasingly costly needs and demands of such 'poverty-stricken' old people. The problems raised by the cuts are central to this book. Financial pressure on local authorities to provide for an increasing number seeking domiciliary services has led them to question their role as to what kind of welfare they should be providing.

Future need for residential and community care services. To summarize, the elderly population is increasing, particularly the very elderly (85+); the numbers of those very disabled or suffering dementia are growing, along with those elderly people living alone. Such groups can be described as vulnerable and likely to need residential care (Willcocks et al, 1987). Table 1.2 shows the need for care among this population.

TABLE 1.2
THE NEED FOR CARE IN GREAT BRITAIN: 1971 - 2001

	1971	1981	1991	2001	1971-2001
Total population ('000's)					% change
Age: 65 - 69	2547	2667	2718	2398	- 9.4
70 - 74	1957	2265	2233	2176	+ 11.2
75 - 79	1301	1601	1793	1825	+ 40.3
80 - 84	773	900	1208	1210	+ 56.6
85+	462	552	843	1047	+126.5

Sources: Adapted from Henwood & Wicks (1986) Table 7 and adjusted on the basis of the following information:

enumerated population, OPCS (1971) Table 6
usually resident population, OPCS (1981) Table 1
1981 based projection for home population - mid year OPCS (1984) Appendix: Table 1

See: Sinclair, I (ed), *Residential care: the research reviewed*, (1988, p.246)

Despite the increasing demand for residential care for the very old (column 5, Table 1.2) and the increasing demand on local authorities to provide an effective package of community care for those expressing a preference to remain in their own environment, this does not necessarily mean an increase in government spending as Ermisch (1983, p.283) demonstrated has been the case over the previous 40 years. There is an underlying assumption in many policy documents that relatives and friends will increase their contribution to care, (for instance, Audit Commission, 1985). As this shows, in a climate of increasing numbers of vulnerable elderly people, the emphasis is on cost-cutting and saving rather than greater emphasis on strategic planning and efficient delivery of services which can meet the needs of individuals (Challis & Davies, 1986).

The total numbers of elderly people have relatively little significance, therefore, in the allocation of resources to services and benefits for the elderly. As Phillipson & Walker in their introduction to *Ageing and social policy* (1986, p.9) state: 'the deciding factors will be political'. The growth of private residential care has indeed demonstrated that the allocation of financial support has been based on an ideology of privatization and anti-state policy rather than on an increase in the numbers of elderly people.

Expenditure on social welfare from 1900 to 1938 grew steadily from under 3 per cent to 11 per cent of Gross National Product. During the 1960's public expenditure accounted for 50 per cent of the national income. Moroney (1976) argues that such a trend in public expenditure can be directly attributed to the increasing role of government in the provision of social services.

TABLE 1.3
PUBLIC EXPENDITURE AND EXPENDITURE ON SOCIAL WELFARE AS PERCENTAGE OF GROSS NATIONAL PRODUCT: 1900-73

Year	Social welfare expenditure	Total public expenditure
1900	2.6	14.4
1910	4.2	12.7
1920	6.8	26.2
1928	9.6	24.2
1938	11.3	30.0
1950	18.0	39.0
1961	17.6	42.8
1968	23.5	52.1
1970	23.7	50.4
1973	24.6	50.5

Sources: Peacock & Wiseman, (1961)
The Growth of Public Expenditures in the U.K.
Tables 9 and 12
National Income & Expenditure. HMSO, 1963-73

See: Moroney, R (1976, p98)

During the 1960's and 1970's the proportion of the nation's resources which was devoted to providing services for elderly people increased seven-fold. In 1953-4 half a per cent of GNP was spent on health and welfare services for old people. By 1979 this figure had risen to two and a half per cent (Thomson, 1984, p.475). Thomson calculates that if:

> the dwindling cash distributions to the elderly are coupled with the massively increased expenditures upon public services for the elderly, a steady rise is recorded in the proportion of the nation's resources being directed towards the elderly. (1984, p.452)

Such a view is not universally shared for others such as Walker (1980) argue that there has been a long period of decline in the resources being allocated to elderly persons. Walker comments:

> Current calls for the trimming of expenditure ... do not succeed a period of wasteful and unsustainable over-pampering of the dependent population in their final years, as too many now seem ready to believe. (1980, p.74)

Although writers such as Walker and Thomson (1984) argue over whether there has been an increase or decrease in expenditure on services for elderly people, it is the changing direction of expenditure toward the private market that dominates the literature of the 1980's. Since 1979, public expenditure has undergone a series of changes. A belief existed that public expenditure was too high and that the welfare state consumed too many resources. Although the government's response to this was to cut expenditure by rolling back the frontiers of the state, it could be argued that they have not been successful in this respect. Robinson (1986, p.3) presents evidence that the level of welfare state expenditure has actually increased between 1979/80 and 1984/85 in respect of both social security (28 per cent) and health and personal social services (17 per cent).

Part of this increase, however, has arisen from the increasing demand, particularly from elderly people for such services and through 'the pursuit of specific policy objectives which led to the unplanned expansion of substitute programmes' (Robinson, 1986, p.19). The state funding of private residential care through the supplementary benefit system could be included here as an example. It can be argued that since 1979 there has not been a *decrease* in expenditure but a *change* in the composition of the expenditure.

Such changes in expenditure in the 1970's and 1980's could be said to herald a new era in the development of welfare - an era of 'residual' state welfare, introducing a retreat of government from the national minimum, curtailment of mass provision on a social need basis and an expansion of support for private provision.

Authors such as Bull & Wilding (1983); Loney (1987); Papadakis & Taylor-Gooby (1987) and Taylor-Gooby (1987) see this period as an abrupt change in the context of the study of state welfare. They would also argue it is the end of a time of agreement and consensus about the role of the state in welfare. Whether there was any consensus is dubious but nevertheless since the 1970's, popular and political confidence in state welfare has withered. Such change has occurred in the context of a number of problems related to the welfare state in the 1960's and 1970's, for example, the rediscovery of poverty and the failure to redistribute resources between the generations (Thomson, 1984).

The 1970's saw the New Right as a major political force arguing that the welfare state was too large, too expensive, too bureaucratic and not very effective in meeting genuine need. The prognosis was that the state should restrict itself to helping only those who could not get support from elsewhere: 'only when the private market and the family broke down should social welfare institutions come into play and then only temporarily' (Titmuss et al, 1974, p.30-31).

Authors such as Golding (1983) describe the moves toward implementing these principles through privatisation, selectivity, and revival of domestication as a return of Victorian values and the 'principles of 1834'.

This argument is weak, however, as the great stance is not one of laissez-faire in relation to private residential care. The private sector as will be seen is held accountable through inspection and regulation and is partly dependent on the public sector for its continued funding. There is also no evidence available to suggest that the family is being thought of as the totally responsible unit. The state has an interest in the well-being of elderly people and their families through policies of county and metropolitan councils. The balance of responsibility between state, family and elderly people is discussed in the next section.

2. Who is responsible for the welfare of elderly people?

1. The elderly person. The popular stereotype of old age as a time of dependency, disability and illness and of reliance on state services is not supported by the facts of ageing (Walker, 1986). Research studies such as Hunt (1978) found that the majority of elderly people were not impaired in any way. The vast majority of elderly people are, therefore, not in need of care and able to look after themselves without help from relatives or social services. Tinker (1984) found that even in residential care the majority were able to dress adequately without supervision. Other writers such as Rossiter & Wicks (1982) and Townsend (1963) found that most people who were unable to care for themselves did not want to be regarded as dependent or have the family give up work to care for them (Salvage, 1988).

Not only are the majority of elderly people looking after themselves, but they provide care for others. Townsend (1963) and Wenger (1984) illustrate the importance of reciprocity in family life, particularly in the role of the elderly person as grandmother. Although the period of retirement is viewed as a time of 'disengagement' (Cumming & Henry, 1961), evidence from numerous studies, particularly those mentioned above, show that elderly people participate in a variety of activities such as Age Concern visiting, political groups and voluntary activities (see Blythe, 1981, p.149 - 152).

Such findings challenge the opinions so often in the literature that elderly people are passive consumers of social services, and dependent on the family.

2. The family. Although the majority of older people are independent, a significant minority are dependent in various ways and require some form of help. Many studies such as Hunt (1978) document the extent to which elderly people are incapacitated and unable to wash, dress or bath themselves. This minority group of 'dependent' elderly people are, however, increasing in number (see section on demography) and questions of who provides and will provide the care are important. A host of studies such as Townsend (1963), and more recently Hunt (1978) and Wenger (1984), illustrate that 'the vast bulk of care is not provided publicly but privately by the family' (Walker, 1985, p.12) and that there are more disabled people living at home and being supported by kinship and friendship networks than there are in institutions.

(a) To what extent is the family responsible for the welfare of older members?

The family still plays a major role in meeting the needs of elderly people (Young & Willmott, 1957; Townsend, 1963; Townsend & Wedderburn, 1965; Rosser & Harris, 1965; Abrams, 1978; Wenger, 1984; Willcocks et al, 1987). Historically, the family as the primary unit of care has been stable despite a variety of false assumptions implicitly embodied in policies which could have unintentionally weakened the family network of care. The constant dilemma, therefore, facing the state is how to support the family to ensure continuity without weakening their responsibility.

Although there is no family policy, there have been policies which effect families and which embody powerful assumptions (Land & Parker, 1978). The state under the Poor Law explicitly assumed that the family had the legal and moral responsibility to meet the needs of its members. It was only when families experienced problems that they were required to place themselves under the care of the state. The family, being a superior institution to the state, should be a private domain, where the state only interferes in special circumstances (Land & Parker, 1978). In some policies this assumption still holds. In others the assumptions are more implicit, for example, it is held that a normal environment for old people consists of a three-generational family, living in close proximity, having strong ties with each other (Townsend, 1963). Another assumption is that the natural role of women within the family, (particularly daughters and daughters-in-law) is to care. This was explicitly set out in the Beveridge Report:

> all women by marriage acquire a new economic and social status with risks and rights different from those of the unmarried ... she undertakes at the same time to perform vital unpaid service. (1942, para. 108)

These assumptions based on research studies such as Townsend above have been embodied in policies where there has been consensus: for example, community care policies which have gone unchallenged by all parties. Although many of the descriptive research studies detailing family life are now dated, the findings are often quoted as valid for the present day situation. The Griffiths Report (1988) embodies some of Townsend's assumptions of family life.

Several trends have challenged these models of the family and 'could reduce effective family support for many elderly people' (DHSS, 1981a, p.59). An increasing number of women have entered the labour force thereby changing their role within and outside the family and also their expectations in relation to responsibilities of care. Trends in divorce and remarriage have thrown doubt on the extended family as the 'normal' structure in family life and families have become more mobile and as a result smaller and less in geographical proximity. All these facts have some impact on the future availability of carers (Walker, 1985). Weir & Simpson (1980) also argue that the ability of the family to provide informal care will be greatly impaired by unemployment and expenditure cuts.

Despite these changes and assumptions embedded in policy, the family has not given up its caring function (Land, 1978; Wicks, 1982; Wright, 1983) or transferred its responsibility to the state (Moroney, 1976). Some even argue that family care has been strengthened (Greengross, 1982).

Others are worried that the family's moral responsibility has declined. Anderson (1971) states that the increasing demand for institutional care indicates a decrease in the family's (or woman's) capacity and willingness to care. Anderson's interpretation of the figures are, however, misleading. Moroney (1976) suggests in relation to public care trends in the 1960's and early 1970's, that the increased rates of admission may not be because of the unwillingness of families to care but a response to the increasing numbers of older people.

(b) Should the family continue to care ?

Research evidence (Land & Parker, 1978; Finch & Groves, 1980; Nissel & Bonnerjea, 1982 and Queshri & Walker, 1986) illustrates that the primary care for elderly people falls increasingly on female relatives often at a high practical and emotional cost. Marxist and feminist writers, such as Henderson (1986) argue that this group continue to bear a disproportionate burden of care, which is reinforced by social policy - particularly policy which keeps people out of institutions and in the community. That women should be prepared to take on such roles and sacrifices, she argues, is not acceptable in the late twentieth century.

While acknowledging this in the feminist literature, few writers go on to prescribe any changes apart from reviewing the prospect of explicit family policy or 'acknowledging the need for a family perspective within the policy-making process' (Wicks, 1987a, p.127).

The alternative view held by traditionalists and conservatives is that it is for families to care for their elderly relatives rather than social services - it is not primarily a state matter. The family is seen as a foundation of a healthy society (Thatcher, 1977). As one commentator states:

> Since the 1970's government publications have increasingly made explicit the ideology of individual responsibility in respect of community care and made crucial to the viability of such care the role of the family. (Henderson, 1986, p.132)

The reality of such statements can be found in *Growing older* (DHSS, 1981a); *A happier old age* (DHSS, 1978) and the Griffiths report (DHSS, 1988).

Despite government intentions to strengthen the responsibility of the family, there are a number of inherent contradictions in their policy. Several studies have found that families who support their dependent relatives are often penalised for so doing. Because of the very fact they are supporting their relatives, services are not provided but resources are steered to those individuals who live alone or who are not supported by family (Hunt, 1970; Davies, 1985). Hunt (1970) found that even when old people moved in with their offspring, services which they previously received were withdrawn.

The incentive for families to look after their elderly relatives is also weakened by the state subsidy enabling elderly people to enter private residential care. It could be argued that the recent idea of a voucher system would avoid this problem by providing people with choice (Minford, 1987); it would also ensure that services were provided in a combination suitable to the user - either pay the family or move into a home.

The whole basis of these assumptions, however, can be questioned because there is no consistent research evidence to support the argument that elderly people turn first to families for help and bureaucratic agencies last.

There is also little evidence that individuals display a coherent set of views toward either the family or the welfare state in terms of who should hold the major responsibility for the care of dependent people. Although the government has drawn a dividing line between formal and informal care (Walker, 1982) in practice:

> the family and welfare state as they are confronted by people in their everyday lives are much less ideological opposites than intermeshed in an overlapping complex of values, needs and interests. (West, 1984, p.417)

In summary, whereas the majority of elderly people are 'independent', the literature portrays them as dependent and in need of care from informal and formal sources. It has been assumed that the former is more important, although little evidence supports this notion. It is not only the concept of the family that has been portrayed in an idealistic light but the idea of community care is also often ill defined in the literature.

(c) Community care

The notion of community care has moved from a narrow definition of the movement out of institutions to domestic settings, to a picture of a caring neighbourhood of family, friends and neighbours or 'gemeinschaft'. Bayley (1973) in the 1970's made the key distinction between care *in* the community and care *by* the community with the notion of the community actually doing the caring.

The 'distorted' view of community care has been emphasised in several government documents such as *Growing old* (DHSS, 1981a) and *A happier old Age*:

> We may need to look increasingly to the wider community to give more support to the kind traditionally expected of the family. (DHSS, 1978)

A more recent document (The Griffiths Report, DHSS, 1988) also appeals to this 'gemeinschaft' notion based on family, friends and neighbours.

There is a danger in much of the writing to conjure up community care as a notion of warmth and kindness yet as a form of social organisation there is little evidence for this. 'The caring community' may not exist. Evandrou, Arber, Dale & Gilbert (1986) found that 'community care for the elderly is only supported with respect to a particular household type - those living alone.' Clarke (1982) also argues that the level of competence necessary to develop and manage an evolving supportive friendship network may be beyond the capacities of many of the dependent people presented as candidates for community care. Although support from friends, neighbours and voluntary bodies is important (Rossiter & Wicks, 1982) what community care really means is care by the family (Equal Opportunities Commission, 1982).

Despite the enthusiasm for community care as a policy and 'priority' there is again little evidence to suggest community care is built around care by neighbours. Outside the personal ties with kin and friends, the responsibilities for others which people acknowledge tend to be narrow and fairly specific, not broad and universal (Bulmer, 1986). Neither has the allocation of resources reflected this commitment in practice. Community care is often seen as a low cost solution, relying on the benevolence of families and their network of informal sources. To maximise this, a notion of shared care or 'partnership' between the state and informal sources of care is promoted and has been voiced in the literature (Barclay Committee, 1982).

In reaction to this Henderson (1986), from a Marxist perspective argues that community care policies have been used on an ideological level to legitimise the reduction or absence of state support.

3. The state. Some writers such as Marshall (1965) and Loney (1987) suggest a consensus existed until the mid 1960's and that 'the overall responsibility for the welfare of citizens remained with the state' (Marshall, 1965, p.97). Others, like Moroney (1976) are doubtful as to whether such consensus ever existed. If it did, it now seems to be breaking down - with disagreement about the state's role and purpose in the welfare arena. The growth of private welfare provision in particular has questioned the role of the state in relation to provision for elderly people.

A residual approach to welfare has been developed by the New Right which is based on the premise that the two natural channels for meeting the individual's needs should be the private market and the family. The state only intervenes when the elderly person can no longer function or has no supportive family. This residual approach has been evident in both the expenditure incurred on welfare services as a whole and on the types of service developed.

Increasingly less attention has been paid in the allocation of resources to the notion of support, with the local authority allocating services to elderly people without families (Moroney, 1976; Hunt, 1978). Resources have also been channelled into services which substitute the family (Moroney, 1976), e.g., into institutional care. In terms of expenditure although the proportion of the nations resources devoted to providing services for elderly people have increased, these have been concentrated on institutional care. The government has increasingly poured money into substituting rather than supporting the family.

The state, however, cannot conceivably afford to take over the total care of the dependent person from the family. Nissel & Bonnerjea, in a small sample calculate that:

> On the assumption that wives and husbands in the sample spent during the complete week on average of between 3 1/2 and 4 hours daily on the care of their relatives, the value of their contribution to the economic output of the country at the rate of £1.80 per hour would have amounted to about £2,500 per family. (1982, p.50)

In recent years the attitude toward the role of the state has changed. Embodied in policy is the assumption that other institutions provide welfare more effectively and that the dismantling of the welfare state is a virtue. By rolling back frontiers of the state, 'the dependency culture' (Walker, 1988) will be overthrown. There is very little empirical evidence to support this. However the present government believes that the role of the state should be an enabling role 'to ensure that domestic policies help to promote self-respect and a sense of individual responsibility' (Walker, 1988, p.17)

As far as elderly people are concerned, the implications have been a reduction of domiciliary services and in institutional state provision. Between 1978 and 1979 and 1983/84 home helps were reduced by 13 per cent, and meals on wheels by 13 per cent to those over 75 (Walker, 1985, p.31). In the same period, the local authority residential care budget per 1000 people aged 75+ was reduced by 30 per cent.

Cost effectiveness has been introduced into criteria being applied to personal social services with disregard for quality. 'Cost effective' however, 'is not the same as care effective' (Walker, 1985, p.31). The language of the private market has entered the public sector and the goal of economic growth and 'enterprise culture' has taken precedence over the goal of welfare. Sections of the literature have latched on to the plight of elderly people in private homes in an attempt to show that profit has overtaken quality of care in welfare provision. Fortunately there is little widespread empirical evidence for such sensationalist reporting.

The state is shown not only to be withdrawing but is 'handing over the welfare of frail elderly people to the insecurities of the market'. Those opposed to such a move believe:

> The outcome will be a two tier system of welfare in which the well-off minority can buy their care freely in the market, while the poor majority will be forced to chose between the inadequate down market elements of the private sector or the residual and under resourced public sector. (Walker, 1985, p.44)

Those advocating a residual approach (Thatcher, 1977) argue that there is less danger of bureaucracy, people would get a better deal and would be able to make proper choice between a variety of options. The role of the state is to ensure that alternative options exist, as Griffiths in the recent community care review states:

> The role of the public sector is essentially to ensure that care is provided. How it is provided is a secondary consideration ... Social services should not be seen as monopolistic providers but arrangers and purchasers of care services. (DHSS, 1988, p.5)

Phillipson (1988) argues that the conclusions of the Griffiths report are flawed by suggesting that the primary role of the state should be one of enabling rather than direct providers of services. Griffiths has 'failed to acknowledge the sociological changes affecting informal care particularly as it relates to older people' (p.22). Phillipson believes that the public sector will maintain a dominant role both in arranging and delivering care services, because community care is not always desirable. He cites research by West (1984) and Salvage (1988) to support his argument to show that families do not provide or want to provide support and that old people feel ambivalent about such support from within the family.

Although Phillipson acknowledges that the state will be more likely to move toward an enabling and facilitating role rather than being a direct provider of care, he ignores the fact that the private sector increasingly fulfils a traditional public sector role as a provider of residential care, and he fails to see that families and public sector agents such as social workers will act as key operators buying into and arranging private care thereby promoting a mixed economy of welfare.

From an alleged consensus position therefore, the literature has become polarised along political lines - with little hardbased evidence to suggest that the state is withdrawing its role in welfare or passing on total responsibility to an effective private market.

3. *Social work and elderly people*

Although elderly people are a significant group in society and in social services terms because of their numbers and their consumption of resources, they are not seen in the literature as a high priority group requiring a social work service. The following section explores the literature to investigate why they are low priority and looks at the role of social work with elderly people.

Elderly people, particularly those over the age of 75, present one of the largest groups in the workload of social services teams (Howe, 1980; Davies, 1985). In Goldberg's (1970) study, although 'the elderly' constituted the largest part of the intake of one local authority area, they made up only a minority of social workers' caseloads. The majority of work with elderly people was carried out by unqualified social work assistants. Despite the creation of a unified social services department in 1971 when work with old people was brought into the mainstream of social work activity and undertaken by generic workers, qualified social workers were still found with caseloads heavily biased toward more prestigious child care cases (Stevenson & Parsloe, 1978; Howe, 1980). Howe found that only 2 per cent of qualified social workers in his study had a bias toward working with elderly and handicapped people, while 91 per cent of all social work assistants had caseloads which were biased in favour of this group.

Social work with elderly people became marginalised within caseloads for a variety of reasons. They were seen as having 'high dependence and low productive potential' (Howe, 1980, p.145). Prevalent in social work attitudes were the stereotypes of ageing - loss and bereavement were seen as natural consequences of ageing, along with 'disengagement' and disease. Many of these concepts were based on early media and sociological research into old age which was very one-sided and negative and has influenced practice to a substantial degree. Social workers found it difficult to identify any positive features in the lives of clients (Brearley, 1975) and many felt there was little chance of effecting change through social work intervention.

As a result, work with elderly people was seen as 'unglamorous' (Black et al, 1983, p.186). The focus of work was on tackling practical problems, responding to requests for help and organising packages of services. Such work was characterised as 'straight forward', 'routine' or even 'casual' (Stevenson & Parsloe, 1978; Black et al, 1983). Black and his colleagues commented:

> It was rare for cases to be seen as being significantly complicated by interpersonal and emotional factors. (1983, p.186)

Phillipson, in a political analysis of ageing found that the unpopularity of work with elderly people was due to 'a range of structural, ideological and organisational factors' (1982, p.104).

Under the present system there are inherent tensions for social workers making their work with elderly people difficult. Economic changes have widened the gap between pensioners and wage earners and cuts in public expenditure have made it difficult to provide facilities to allow old people to remain in the community.

Social work with elderly people is also restricted because legislation is weighted toward children and families. There is some evidence (The Barclay Committee report of 1982) that teams bombarded with referrals engage only in legislative work. Preventative work, particularly with elderly people is lost and social work with elderly people becomes of 'marginal' significance.

Finally, the academic environment has done little in the past to promote 'a critical perspective' on older people in the welfare state. Child care research has been seen as academically more stimulating and for those seeking radical therapies, involvement with older people was judged to constitute a form of professional or political suicide (Phillipson, 1982, p.107).

Academic studies have also concentrated on social work in a generic setting. Very few have focused on teams working exclusively with elderly people or on practice rather than service orientated approaches such as reality orientation with dementia sufferers. Although such studies exist in other literature, few have been researched in social work settings.

Gerontological literature must also take the blame for reinforcing this. There has been little criticism of existing literature and many of the studies, as quoted above, only serve to reinforce the negative image of old age. There is also little evidence that the emerging radical perspectives in social work literature have influenced actions toward elderly people in any way.

The role and function of social work with elderly people. A review of the practical social work literature reveals a lack of clarity in the aims and roles of social work with elderly people.

Historically there has been a shift from an administrative role, hinging mainly around individual applications to residential care, to a casework and assessment role (Means & Smith, 1985; Townsend, 1962). This movement was partly due to the need, by medical social workers, to use casework models of intervention to work through 'the fears and feelings of disability' in old age. There was also an increasing need for assessment of elderly people particularly in relation to emotional and relationship problems prior to their admission into residential care and especially as a number were having to wait at home for an available placement.

Although the literature portrays casework and counselling on an individual basis as one of the predominant areas of social work with elderly people (Reid & Epstein, 1972; Goldberg & Warburton, 1979; The Barclay Committee, 1982; Phillipson, 1982; Black et al, 1983), there are other functions which could be described as central to the social work task with elderly people.

In 1977 The British Association of Social Workers emphasised the areas of work most appropriately dealt with by the qualified social worker. They can be summarised as :

a) assessing need;

b) providing skilled social work help with problems of relationship, problems arising from crises, loss, change or other social, emotional or medical condition;

c) providing the skill in helping to overcome psychological problems related to recurring practical, financial and advocatory help;

d) providing group and community work;

e) understanding and accepting the degree of risk which the client is prepared to take and balancing this with the sometimes over- anxious reaction of society;

f) enabling and supporting others in caring;

g) participating in planning and policy making related to elderly people.

Although there is potential for developing social work with elderly people in these areas, the 'maintenance' function of social workers in work with elderly people has been widely confirmed by Glendenning (1981); Sainsbury (1981); Black et al (1983) and Davies (1985). In three-quarters of the cases found by Goldberg & Warburton (1979, p.93) the 'preservation of the status quo was all the social worker was hoping for'.

Although this has been questioned as a 'proper' and 'effective' function of social work (Goldberg et al, 1978), possibly more suited to the task of volunteers and community networks, such maintenance and surveillance are now:

> perhaps the major area of concern because of the high costs of meeting illness and disability among the increasing numbers of old. (Means & Smith, 1985, p.364)

Other 'common' elements in the social work role with elderly people highlighted by the literature include the social worker as mobiliser of domiciliary and residential resources (Black et al, 1983; Bowl, 1986); as a co-ordinator of services, particularly with the increasing emphasis on partnership with 'communities' and their networks through community care schemes (Challis & Davies, 1980); and the social worker as a monitor of services (Barclay Committee, 1982).

More recent research on effectiveness has been applied to settings with elderly people. Challis & Davies (1980) and Davies & Challis (1986) in their research monitor the effectiveness of community care packages and as a result show more effective ways of deploying social work resources in line with their clients needs. This has been achieved with the social worker carrying responsibility for a budget. Unfortunately although these schemes, for example, the Kent Community Care Scheme (Challis & Davies, 1986) are widely publicised through the popular social work literature, they have not been compared or widely applied in practice.

The Barclay Committee (1982) see the 'unique' role for social workers as coordinators in social care planning, but this view has been challenged by some who see the role of other social service workers as more important. Means & Smith (1985) in their review of historical developments of welfare services conclude that home help organisers through their closer day to day contact with families and neighbourhood are more appropriate to play a more direct role in the allocation of all domiciliary services. Dexter & Harbert (1983) in *The home help service* argue that they should be seen clearly as head of the domiciliary team, with the social worker only entering the scene when specialist skills are required.

The evidence is clear, however, that the social worker acting as a resource person about networks, communities and services, strengthens the roles of home helps, wardens and ancillaries (Hadley, 1981; Goldberg & Connelly, 1982). In recent years another key function has appeared in the literature with increasing emphasis - the social worker as gatekeeper to services. This is closely allied to the role of the social worker in rationing resources (Black et al, 1983). It could be argued that this gatekeeping function is an uncomfortable role as it creates a tension for social workers on the one hand attempting to carry out a bureaucratic role and on the other attempting to meet the need of each elderly person.

The Barclay Committee would disagree:

> We do not accept the argument that this is not a part of the social work role, although we sympathise with the social worker's distaste for it ... we may have as our aim a service available to all in need, but we need it to be quietly rationed. (1982, p.109)

Phillipson (1982) argues that to accept this stance of the social worker just providing services and support in the existing system will lead social work into 'a blind alley'. He advocates a more radical approach to the problems of old age. Although legislation empowering social workers to act points directly to the needs of individual clients rather than communities (Black et al, 1983) an increasingly important role for the social worker is in improving the general lot of elderly people. A more political oriented literature - attempting to raise the political status of elderly people can only be seen as positive. This view, however, is not shared by other writers in the field.

Others, such as Rowlings (1981) feel that advocacy on behalf of elderly people in terms of welfare rights, housing and finance should not be the concern of social workers. It is also argued that social workers employed as agents of the state should take existing political, economic and social structures and policy as given and carry out the tasks for which they were employed - counselling those in need to help them adapt to the situation in which they find themselves (Barclay Committee, 1982, p.110). Yet very often personal and structural problems are intertwined and the social worker has no choice but to determine a 'political role'. The appropriateness of such a role within the boundaries of a public sector agency however, have not been questioned in the literature relating to elderly people.

In conclusion, this section shows that the literature has been dominated by the provision of social services to elderly people rather than any practice based focus. The relatively little documentation on practice issues with elderly people reflects the low priority given to work with elderly people among fieldwork teams.

This is also due to the lack of clarity in the social work role - an issue which has not yet been addressed in the gerontological literature. Neither the appropriate role of the social worker working as a public sector agent with elderly people nor their role in other arenas of welfare such as the private sector has been discussed.

The development of residential care for elderly people

Historical overview from 1834 onwards

An historical overview of residential care during this period illustrates the ad hoc development of public services for elderly people and highlights the lack of a conceptual framework for residential care in relation to other public services and other welfare sectors. Although residential care accommodates relatively few elderly people and has been viewed in the literature as 'the last resort', it is surprising that it has dominated the history of welfare provision and policy for elderly people for so long.

The original role of residential care following the 1834 Poor Law Amendment Act was to act as a deterrent by way of applying the principle of 'less eligibility' to those seeking indoor relief:

> Those who were to be given relief should not be able to experience conditions of life as good as, or better than those experienced by the independent labourer of the lowest class. (Townsend, 1962, p.20)

It was only with the 1948 National Assistance Act that residential care was viewed as more than a housing provision. The Act was a significant landmark in the history of welfare provision for elderly people. It abolished the Poor Law, singled out elderly people as a separate category and disassociated their needs (McCoy, 1986). It also placed a duty on local authorities to provide:

> Residential accommodation for persons who by reason of age, infirmity or any other circumstances are in need of care and attention not otherwise available to them. (1948 National Assistance Act, Section 21)

The definition of 'in need of care and attention' was to change the focus of residential care from merely a provision of shelter to the provision of welfare including the concepts of welfare such as food, bodily care, health care, care for disabled, etc. In this sense the Act contained real substantive reform. This also applied to the financial arrangements.

Welfare authorities were not only to provide accommodation (known as Part III accommodation) but would charge an 'economic rent' for them so that any old person who wished to go into a home could do so in exactly the same way as people accustomed to going into residential hotels. Financially independent elderly people entered residential care, paid a full economic charge and were cared for alongside people with no income or capital other than a supplementary pension (Gill, 1988).

The optimism embodied in this Act, however, did not materialise in practice. The hotel simile proved to be unrealistic. Pensions did not provide enough for elderly people to meet the economic rent and an element of need for care rather than choice was evident. It was also not available on demand as envisaged. The Act was contradictory in that it defined residential care as a 'caring' provision, yet proposed a new form of residential care - to be run on a hotel model. Such a model, however, did not transpire for frail, elderly people.

The increasing pressure on accommodation by increasing numbers in the elderly population and the restrictions on capital investment made it difficult to close the old institutions and build the new smaller homes envisaged by the Nuffield Foundation in 1944. Well into this century, therefore, public sector residential care operated in old poor law buildings and employed staff who had worked within the poor law system.

The lack of direction in policy for residential care was not only evident in capital investment, but also in the design of new residential homes. Real improvements in the quality of care were also few and far between. Such was the situation in the late 1950's when Townsend reported:

> The great majority of residents live in poor conditions. A large number of residents sleep in rooms containing more than 10 or 20 beds. Most residents are obliged to sit, eat and sleep in 1 of 3 large rooms and sometimes all 3 functions are served by one room. The matrons and wardens wield considerable power. Few of the residents wear their own clothes. Religious and social activities are organised. (Townsend, 1962, p.107)

The Act could have gone a lot further to improve the plight of elderly people if everything embodied in it had been put into practice. It fell far short of expectations and did not result in better conditions for all elderly people. This was partly because it left confusion about the distinction between elderly people who were sick and those in the need of care and attention. It also failed in its objective because of its almost total reliance on residential care.

Beyond this Act little thought was put into the needs and demands of elderly people. In welfare provision as a whole, therefore, residential care remained 'severely underconceptualised' (Willcocks, 1987, p.20). Institutions did nothing to address the problems of physical and mental infirmity commonly associated with old age, but merely maintained those people who couldn't look after themselves at home but were not considered ill enough to go into hospital.

Because of a lack of rationale for residential care in relation to welfare provision as a whole, piecemeal developments have followed in residential care services. The lack of co-ordination and strategic planning with other sectors has led to a decrease in public sector residential care and an increase and duplication in provision by other sectors. It is not surprising that alternative private sector provision has emerged when public sector residential care is still viewed as a 'last resort', devalued by professionals and clients and still contains elements of the workhouse system. The result can be described as a 'crisis' within residential care - to the extent that a radical revision of the purpose and nature of residential care is called for.

Three related issues, however, dominated the 1950's and 1960's which eventually led to the promotion of alternative provision and questioned the role of residential care in the spectrum of services for elderly people.

1. Restrictions in local authority capital building meant that only the really frail and infirm elderly with a need entered residential care.

Rationing systems developed and the idea of residential care for active elderly people was abandoned under the pressure of demand.

2. The high cost of hospital care, and the growth of NHS day hospitals meant that people who previously would have been inpatients could live in old peoples homes and go to hospital as outpatients.

3. Related to this was the continuing lack of clarity in the definition 'in need of care and attention', which shifted to include highly dependent people suffering incontinence, serious loss of mobility and 'abnormal' senile dementia. Criteria had to be developed to determine respective responsibilities between home and hospital because of such overlapping dependency. However, the dividing responsibility for the care of dependent elderly people between health and social services created a distinction which in practice was meaningless as elderly people entered care because of a combination of both medical and social factors (Sinclair, 1988).

In addition to problems of definition, the 1960's heralded a series of studies and reports that highlighted the disadvantages of residential care and questioned its very existence. Townsend (1962) in particular, produced in *'The Last Refuge'* a mass of evidence portraying the misery of institutional life. This became a landmark in the development of attitudes to old peoples homes and demonstrated the failure of the state to end public assistance institutions after 1948. Not only Townsend (1962) but Goffman (1961) writing on *'Asylums'* and Miller & Gwynne (1972) in relation to institutions for handicapped and chronically sick people, challenged the attitudes and philosophy underlying residential care.

These three, together with other specific studies related to elderly people, for example, *Sans everything* (Robb, 1967) and *Taken for a ride* (Meacher, 1972), a study of elderly mentally confused people - all focused on the relationship and personality within residential care. The main conclusion was that institutions were cut off from mainstream society and were not representative of family life in any way.

Much of the academic writing of such left wing sociologists condemning the public sector has had long term and severely damaging consequences for future public sector provision. Not only did the sociologists of the time undermine the power of the public sector by theoretical errors, concentrating on the institution and not its inhabitants, but they provided a negative critique without any suggestion of an alternative.

At the time despite the condemnation of institutional life spelt out in these studies there was a feeling of complacency (Means & Smith, 1985). Residential care was still seen as the most economic provision for elderly people, particularly as increasing numbers of elderly people placed a burden on the pension system.

Positive government reviews of residential care also reinforced the usefulness of residential care as a provision for elderly people. Harris reported:

> The gloomy picture of old people's homes being inhabited by masses of

unhappy discontented residents is not supported by any evidence from this inquiry. (Harris 1968, p.69)

Parallel to the production of critical literature, much of the writing of the late 1950's and 1960's, records a change in attitude and thinking about services for elderly people. Welfare for old people was said to have moved to become a preventative service, enabling people to remain at home through the expansion of domiciliary services, such as home help provision and meals-on-wheels, thus reducing the need for admission into residential care. In such ways local authorities were concerned to promote the welfare of all old people rather than simply cater for the minority needing residential care (Brown, 1972). The research and literature on community care, however, initially had very little widespread impact on developments. Although the community initiatives such as Kent Community Care schemes were - and continue to be - well documented, their arguments have not been strong enough to ensure widespread application and most have remained local initiatives.

Two studies - *The aged in the welfare state* (Townsend & Wedderburn, 1965) and *Old people in three industrial societies* (Shanas et al, 1968) - stressed the need for an expansion of domiciliary services, yet there still existed the underlying assumption that families should care for their elderly relative and a concern as to whether domiciliary services undermined the willingness of families to care. Although other studies, for example, *The family life of old people* (Townsend, 1963), show that this was not true, residential care continued to dominate the welfare scene.

Developments since 1970. Considerable emphasis on a preventative approach was taken a step further in 1971 with the reorganisation of personal social services following the Seebohm Report (Seebohm Committee, 1968) which attempted to rationalize a fragmented system into a single Social Services Department led by social workers. Although this brought work with old people into the mainstream of social work activity, it can be argued that it did not create the organizational structure necessary to keep elderly people at risk in the community.

Hadley & Hatch (1981) argue that the new departments did not have adequate resources such as home helps, or have systems to give early knowledge of those at risk. As a result public sector residential care remained the major provision for elderly people. Means and Smith (1985) argue that this was also due to three factors: trade union and professional self interest; the symbolic importance of institutions and the continuing concern about hospital costs. However, although there is some justification for these arguments, residential care remained the dominant provision because many welfare professionals believed that frail and sick elderly people could only adequately be cared for in such settings. The views of elderly people themselves were somewhat neglected.

Residential care also dominated state provision because of the failure of domiciliary services to supersede it. The adverse economic climate and the start of public expenditure cuts in the mid-1970's affected local authority domiciliary services. Although the priorities document of the DHSS (1976) led the government to decide on a 2 per cent increase in domiciliary services and a decrease in residential accommodation to account for it, the expansion in packages of care to enable people to remain at home did not materialise. Residential care was seen as the 'last resort' (DHSS, 1981a) with care of elderly people transferred to the community (DHSS, 1978; DHSS, 1981b) but the intention did not become real. The Audit Commission (1985) reported in conclusion that the variation between local authority spending on residential and community care did not reflect political choices made between the two, since authorities spending little on residential care spent little also on community care. No commitment, therefore has been made to a community care alternative. This again points to a lack of co-ordinated development of service and the confusion and uncertainty around the function and purpose of old peoples homes in the modern welfare state (Gill, 1988).

The purpose and nature of residential care has, however, changed. It has moved further away from being an accommodation need alone to a caring need and a more positive approach has been taken with a move toward the concerns of elderly people themselves including their individual emotional as well as physical needs.

The function of residential care as viewed in the literature has broadened; new facilities have been developed, an attempt has been made to integrate homes into the community, and residential care has become multi-functional and part of a network of resources to help people to remain in their own homes. In 1981 a survey of residential accommodation for elderly people was undertaken by the Personal Social Services Research Unit. They found that 75 per cent of local authority homes provided day care within the home and 11 per cent had attached day centres. The concept of short term care was introduced in 1967 and acted as relief care for relatives or helped elderly people to convalesce after a hospital stay. Eighty-one per cent of homes were also found to provide day care and short term stays along with meals-on-wheels (Darton, 1986).

It can be argued that some of these additions have come about in order to improve the image of public sector care. Many of these functions, however, have not been fully integrated conceptually into overall provision and as a result residential care is still viewed in the literature as a provision after all else fails.

Also, developments to prevent admission were not necessarily viewed as a good thing. Allen (1983) questioned whether traditional local authority homes were the right environment for such resource centres and others, such as Challis & Davies (1986), have pointed to the problems caused by the fragmentation and lack of co-ordinated and strategic planning of domiciliary and residential provision.

Developments in the late 1970's and early 1980's have again focused increasingly on the standard and quality of care in residential homes, not only in an attempt to improve their image but also to go some way in reflecting the demands and needs of its 'consumers'.

The literature reported above, can be criticised for placing emphasis on aspects of environmental determinism and effects of institutional life rather than on a concern for the rights of residents themselves and as a result has hampered the development of important concepts such as privacy and autonomy. The focus on these issues increasingly comes from a consumer perspective.

With the development of alternative sectors of care, comparisons based on 'effectiveness', 'efficiency' and 'economics' have permeated the literature on residential care over the last decade.

Although this approach to welfare is 'not simply a by-product of contemporary monetarist ideology' (Judge, Knapp & Smith, 1986, p.113), as contracting out to other sectors has been a frequent feature over a number of years, the search for value for money and efficiency in the production of welfare has predominated many studies to a greater extent than ever before: for instance, Judge (1985) and the Audit Commission report, 'Making a reality of Community Care' (1986).

An evaluation of cost-effectiveness by looking at resource inputs (eg. Home help services) and outputs has been developed in the 'production of welfare model' (Davies & Knapp, 1981; Knapp, 1984; Davies 1986). A similar model relating to quality of residential care has been a valuable contribution to the literature on the economics of residential care, and had been widely applied. As a result of its application, private provision of residential care is described as 'good value for money' (Judge, 1985). There is a danger, however, in comparing sectors on the basis of economic factors alone, without looking at the wider ethical, social and consumer perspectives.

1988 onwards: a challenge for the 1990s

1. Residential care as a positive choice and experience

Residential care is often seen as the last resort following the failure of support to enable people to remain at home. It is argued that a change in perspective is necessary so that elderly people can view residential care as a 'positive choice':

> We believe that people should be able to make a positive choice between different models of care, when they can no longer cope with life unaided. At present they are too often presented with a stark choice between remaining in the community and moving into residential care. We believe that if needs for services and accommodation are looked at separately, however, the range of possible choice for each individual can be vastly expanded. (Wagner Report, 1988, p.3)

The choice not only exists between community and residential care but between different sectors of residential care, particularly a choice between private and public sector care.

2. The local authority as co-ordinator, not sole provider

The role of the local authority in relation to residential care is changing. Care in an institutional setting as it has evolved over the last century and a half may cease as local authorities relinquish their role as the dominant providers of care. Griffiths (DHSS, 1988) argues that local authorities should be given greater responsibility for running community care and 'ensure that care is provided. How it is provided is an important but secondary condition' (DHSS, 1988 p.5).

Local authorities will therefore become organisers, designers and purchasers rather than direct providers of service.

In reviewing the historical development of residential care this appears a radical departure from the traditional role of the public sector in residential care provision, which until the early 1980's remained the dominant provider.

It is not surprising, however, that such a junction has been reached in the future direction of residential care services. The public sector, despite its attempts to improve its image and develop a coherent rationale for residential care, has a bad track record in introducing changes and including consumer views in its process of change. The literature of the 1960's clearly and damagingly reinforced the image of residential care as the last resort and devalued it as a caring provision, without providing an alternative model. Sociologists of the time failed to see the implications of their actions, which in some ways ensured the limited survival of public sector domination in residential care provision.

Residential care and social work

In relation to residential care for old people there appears to be a lack of clarification in the social work role (Rowlings, 1981). Residential social work, described as the extension of the worker/client relationship in a residential setting is about:

> working with people in a shared day-to-day living experience and applies to areas of the client's life not ordinarily shared by a social worker. (Ward, 1980)

The role of the field social worker as described by the literature therefore concentrates on outside activity and is seen as separate. Whether in practice this distinction can be maintained is questionable. Interaction across the boundary is, however, a core activity in any form of residential intervention aiming to enable people to cope more effectively in their new environment (Ward, 1980; Booth, 1985; Willcocks et al, 1987). It is at the boundary that the roles of field and residential social worker meet. This review looks at the process of admission from the perspective of the field social worker and looks at their function up to and beyond the boundary of residential care.

Assessment of the need for residential care. Because residential care places in the public sector are not available on demand, the social worker is engaged in rationing and allocating this scarce resource. This involves an assessment of the client based on their need and the risks they face as well as the availability of the resource (Curnock & Hardiker, 1979).

Townsend in *The last refuge* (1962) described the assessment process as speedy and essentially 'a superficial examination of the facts, without thorough inquiry into the alternatives' (Townsend 1962 p.129). This is now an out of date perception as practice has fortunately moved on and a variety of assessment models are in use.

Assessment of the individual's suitability for residential care is however, problematic because it is based on the social worker's professional judgement of each individual's different circumstances - in other words there are no hard scientific criteria against which to measure the risks. This introduces an element of social work autonomy into the decision-making process.

Considering the difficulties faced in a professional assessment together with the fact that the majority of people who enter private residential care do not use the services of a social worker (Willcocks et al, 1987) and are in general adequately placed, i.e., in need of residential care (Bradshaw & Gibbs, 1987a) the role of the social worker may be redundant.

Supporting this argument are the many examples of shortcomings in social work assessment (Neill, 1982), the overlap in characteristics of residents in relation to other provision (Plank, 1977; Wilkin & Jolley, 1979) and the inappropriateness of placements (Smith & Lowther, 1976; Brocklehurst et al, 1978; Ovenstone & Bean, 1981). Such inappropriate admissions illustrated by these authors may be due in part to the lack of clarity in the purpose of residential care and also to the changing needs of elderly people seeking care.

In the view of Wagner, the nominated social worker should be acting as the agent of the potential user to procure the services of which he or she is in need, and in assessment:

> The social worker must primarily regard themself as the agent of the user and be recognised as such by the management of the providing agency. (Wagner 1988, p.28)

The assessment role is clearly seen by Wagner as part of the social work task:

> The primary responsibility to carry out an assessment of the capabilities and disabilities of the individual and of eligibility for the service lies with the social worker ... and each individual family should have available to them the skills of a nominated social worker in order to carry out the assessment. (Wagner 1988, p.28)

Based on an individual assessment of need, the report advocates that the social worker should be able to identify alternatives available to the user, and to ensure the individual has clear and realistic information about these. This involves the use of social work skills in new ways particularly in the creation of packages of care.

The underlying danger here, however, exists when the social worker raises expectations that the agency cannot reach. Enhanced choice only exists when resources are available, accessible and acceptable. Studies have shown that residential care is often not easily acceptable and is not selected out of personal choice but often as the result of the decisions of others (Neill et al, 1986; Willcocks et al, 1987).

The role of the social worker, therefore, lies mainly in making the stages of admission (arranged by other members of the family or a professional) less painful (Davies, 1985).

Stages in the process of admission. The deleterious effects of the process of becoming a resident have been well documented (Goffman, 1961; Miller &

Gwynne, 1972; Parkes, 1972; Tobin & Lieberman, 1976; Norman, 1980). Tobin and Lieberman write:

> The grey portrait, which has been attributed to actually living in an institutional environment, can be understood as the end stage of a process that begins well before entering and living in these facilities. The earliest period in the process even precedes the decision to seek institutional care ... Another identifiable period follows the decision to seek care and another when the person is waiting entrance into the institution. The first two months after entering is the initial adjustment phase and by the end of the year, the resident has either adapted to the institution and survived intact or has deteriorated or died. (Tobin & Lieberman 1976, p.21)

In adapting the work of Goffman, Jones (1972) outlines four main stages in the process; each stage having implications for the role and tasks faced by the social worker.

1. Preparation

This is the waiting period before admission takes place and has been described as a time which 'leaves the prospective resident feeling abandoned and rejected prior to any action' (Tobin & Lieberman, 1976).

Research by Willcocks et al (1987) shows that residents are better able to come to terms with anticipating admission when they had experienced some control over the process. The social worker should therefore involve the elderly person at each stage of the plan and keep them informed of all decisions and their implications. In reality, however, few prospective residents have knowledge of what will happen in the process or of what the residential home will be like prior to their arrival (Shaw & Walton, 1979). Yet as Parkes comments: the more information that they have about the world into which they are moving, the less chance there is of misunderstanding, confusion and personal distress arising (Parkes 1972, p.224).

2. Separation

Separation from close relatives is the second stage in the process - one which is often accompanied by illness (Brearley, 1975). Pope (1978), in a study in South Glamorgan found that of emergency admissions 12.2 per cent died within the first three months.

From notification to the time of admission the social worker may be involved in casework involving reminiscence work and bereavement counselling connected to leaving home and family. This may also involve working with the feelings and anxieties of others, for example daughters who are involved in the admission.

3. Transition

Research by Pope (1978) shows that other people taking decisions for the elderly person and the practices related to admission - such as loss of a pension book - may not only increase dependency but reinforce to the new resident the separateness of the resident from community life. It is here that the boundaries between field and residential social workers meet. During this time social workers should be seen as an integral part of the care team, linking and liaising with residential staff to design care plans and to prepare a contract together with the resident.

4. Incorporation

This marks the ending of one phase and the beginning of another in institutional care, when the social worker undertakes to help elderly people establish new relationships with residents and staff. At this stage, it is important to pause and reflect back on the opening paragraph of this section acknowledging the distinction between field and residential social work. Although this chapter has chosen to view them separately, the whole discussion about the extent to which residential care is a social work activity is central to this thesis. A number of CCETSW papers (for instance, Paper No. 3, 1973) proposed unified training for field and residential staff and clearly see residential care providing a social work service. The question of appropriate staff and training to carry out such a function has again been raised with the increasing numbers of frail elderly people requiring staff with relevant nursing qualifications. The emphasis in the private sector has been on the latter function with a neglect very often of the residents social care arrangements (Weaver, 1985b). This, therefore has implications for the social work role in the private sector of care.

One body of literature therefore, describes the social worker in an active role in the process, ideally ensuring that the elderly person has choice, control and can exercise self determination.

Variables in the process of admission. Public sector literature reveals that not only the characteristics of elderly people but also the processes leading to allocation and admission are important in an understanding of how and why people enter residential care.

Mitchell & Earwicker conclude that:

> The decision to allocate is the result of complex interactions between an applicant's characteristics and circumstances, the context of the allocation meeting(s) and the procedures, processes and inter-participant dynamics of the allocation meeting. (Mitchell & Earwicker 1982, p.57)

1. Client variables

Despite numerous research attempts it is impossible to draw a picture of a typical successful applicant for a residential home. However, there is evidence of a selection bias: that is, particular kinds of people enter residential care (Tobin & Lieberman, 1976; Willcocks et al, 1986; Barnes, 1980; Cooper, 1985; Hughes & Wilkin, 1980). These studies find that people newly admitted to homes tend to be very old (on average aged 83), predominantly female, and single - often through widowhood.

The majority of people who apply for residential care, however, do so less from choice than from circumstances (Neill et al, 1988), many applicants being reluctant to enter a home (Sinclair, 1986). The circumstances under which people enter care are also very varied and often reflect an accumulation of problems. Sinclair et al (1988) found that those who entered local authority homes were on average older, more disabled and more likely to have high cognitive impairment scores than the rest of the sample of old people living alone. In a recent article, Sinclair et al (1988) also provide a very useful attempt at predicting the social, physical and cognitive factors leading to admission, through a technique which can be widely and usefully applied. The collapse in existing support systems also provides a main group of reasons for admission (Mitchell & Earwicker, 1982; Willcocks et al, 1982) particularly if this involves looking after a confused elderly person (MacLennan et al, 1984).

2. Context variables

Along with the lack of informal support, inadequate domiciliary support and inadequate housing are found to precipitate admission (Townsend, 1962) sometimes unnecessarily (Harris, 1968; Bradshaw and Gibbs, 1987b). Such studies identifying elderly people vulnerable to residential care are vital if the policy is to keep people at home for as long as possible.

The success of admission into local authority residential care depends also on matters outside the individual's control: for example, resources, policies of social services department and skills of the social worker presiding over the case (Neill, 1982). Allocation of a place is often a political decision based on resource availability and variation (Mitchell & Earwicker, 1982) and influenced more by logistics than client need (Davies, 1985).

Because of such shortfall in local authority provision potential residents often find themselves in homes other than their preferred choice, having gone through a decision-making process where they had very little personal choice (Wilding, 1983). Neill et al found that the problem of providing choice did not arise primarily from the disabilities of the old people in their study or the strains of the carers:

> Choice was constrained because of the context within which the application was made - a hospital or a home of a relative who was unwilling to continue to provide care. (Neill 1988, p.194)

Previous happenings also influenced the context in which the decision was taken (Mitchell & Earwicker, 1982). McCoy (1983) found that in Suffolk the suitability of an applicant for a vacancy in a particular home, depended on the level of dependency of other residents and the ability of the home to deal with such dependency.

3. Process variables

Paterson (1978) argues that the processes of selection are important in determining who is allocated a residential home place.

Although the definition of 'urgency' varies, the concept is often a consideration in sorting out clients. Neill (1982) found there was a pressure on social workers to define their client's situation in crisis terms in order to obtain a local authority vacancy.

It is not only emergency placements that 'befoul the system', (Neill, 1982, p.235) but there is also evidence of the allocation process being by-passed through the 'swop' system (Davies, 1979). Residents in hospital - who were not in need of hospital nursing care but who were too 'frail' to return home - were often swopped with residents in residential homes who 'needed' hospital attention. Neill (1982) supports Davies's finding and suggests that the process of admission from hospital was different because residential homes were used as a dumping ground by some consultants.

There is other evidence that hospitalization precipitates applications, (Neill et al, 1988). Clough, (1981) & Paterson, (1978) suggest that the need to clear hospital beds, the reluctance of relatives to resume the burdens of caring or their anxieties about an old person's safety combine with the old person's frailty and loss of confidence to produce the belief that residential care is the only option for a particular hospital patient.

This has vast implications for the process of admission because a higher than average proportion of old people are in hospital when they apply (Bebbington & Tong, 1983; Stapleton, 1976).

The explicit aim of residential care - that is, to provide care and attention - may, therefore, be questioned. Hospital patients may need considerable care and attention, while the local authority may attempt to liken their home to the original conception of a hotel (Neill, 1982). As a result elderly people may be placed inappropriately.

How the case is presented at the allocation meeting and discussed is again highlighted as an important component of the process of admission. Attributes of individual social workers and the chairmen of such meetings are important in influencing whether a place is obtained (Mitchell & Earwicker, 1982).

The process of decision-making, however, varies widely and may not be a panel decision, but one taken centrally by a social worker in consultation with her senior. But even where allocation panels exist:

> The only characteristic which all these 16 panels seemed to have in common was that a group of people met on a regular basis to discuss a Part III application. Other than this, the composition of panels, their stated roles and function and their authority as a group to make decision and take action showed wide variation. (Neill 1982, p.239)

In reviewing the process, Billis describes it as:

> A web of interwoven decisions, not beginning from one point and progressing steadily towards an end result but taken simultaneously in a number of different corners of the department. (Billis 1973, p.455)

Literature on the social work role in residential care does not go very far to clarify the complexities in the decision-making process of admission, the one main conclusion is that the role of the social worker in the public residential care system is not clear cut. Although one of their main tasks may be of assessment, allocation of residential placements are less likely to be based on assessed needs of clients than on the needs of the organisation which social workers, as agents of the public sector, reflect in their practice of assessment and admission to residential care.

This illustrates one of the distortions in the attempt to match resident with home. Little research has focused on this or on one of the other major distortions - the social worker operating in a situation of market forces.

The growth of the private sector

The recent debates on the role of residential care (Audit Commission, 1985; The Wagner Report, 1988 and The Firth Report, DHSS, 1987b) have emerged not only as a result of increasing numbers of elderly people and the pressure on public expenditure or the unease that elderly people are victims of unacceptable standard of care, but also because of the substantial growth of private residential care.

Although the literature marks 1980 as a time of a boom in private residential care provision, the history of private care goes back a long way and 'from some perspectives private welfare is a reality whose time is past' (Papadakis & Taylor-Gooby, 1987, p.2). The growth in private care, therefore is not only an artifact of current political ideology (Kellaher, 1988).

The private sector as a major provider of residential care for elderly people was however late in arriving. Until the 1970's the state provided the majority of residential places with private residential care being used as an extension of state provision if someone required specialist care.

Since the late 1970's, however, there has been a massive growth of the private residential sector as Diagram 1.1 illustrates. Although there is a north-south divide in provision (Larder, Day & Klein, 1986), Suffolk has been one of the major areas of private sector expansion. Between 1976 and 1981 there was a 50 per cent growth in the numbers of residents in private homes while local authority residential provision grew in the same period by only 6 per cent (McCoy, 1984). While the private residential provision is expanding at an exponential rate the local authority is at a standstill. It is not surprising, therefore, that the private sector has emerged as an alternative to state provision, given the criticism of public sector provision by sociologists of the 1960's, which undermined the power of that sector without providing an adequate alternative.

However, reasons for expansion are also found among a number of demographic and social changes which have taken place. Among such reasons, are increasing numbers of elderly people, the closure of long stay hospital institutions and decreasing numbers of available carers to care for such discharged patients, all which have coincided with a period of public sector cutbacks. Ratecapping has meant that local authorities have less resources to channel into residential provision and as 'community care' is the preferred policy, scarce resources are channelled in this direction. As a result public residential care has remained static.

On the other hand, private residential care has boomed making up for a shortfall in geriatric beds and in local authority care. Gill (1988) found a strong inverse correlation between local authority provision and private and voluntary provision - and concludes that in areas where the provision of local authority and health authority residential services is relatively low, there is a flourishing private sector, irrespective of the level of need for residential services from area to area.

Also accounting for the growth in private residential care is the government's ideological commitment to privatisation. This was put into practice through the supplementary benefit system with large amounts of public money funding the private sector.

DIAGRAM 1.1
RESIDENTIAL ACCOMMODATION FOR PERSONS AGED 65 YEARS AND OVER IN ENGLAND (1976-1987)

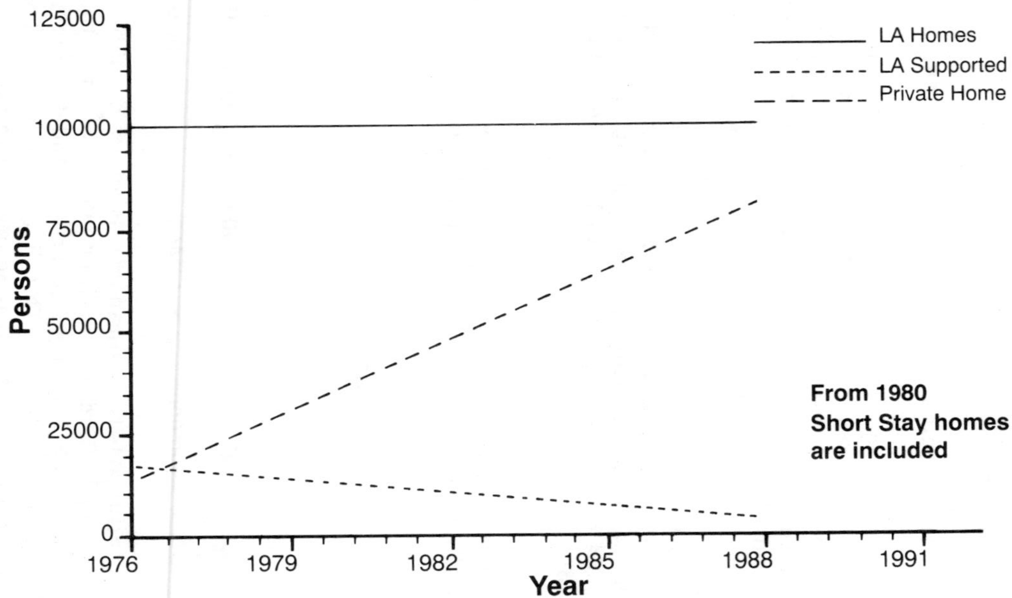

Source: Based on figures provided by HMSO (1987) Health & Personal Social Services Statistics for England, 1987 Ed. DHSS (1987 figures are provisional)

Kellaher et al, (1988, p.8)

Whether the implications for private residential care of the change in regulations relating to board and lodgings allowance were accidental and unforseen or whether the changes had been designed to encourage privatisation is debatable. Walker (1986, p.30) believes that the move was primarily 'a matter of ideology'. However, the haphazard nature of such changes in funding does suggest it was an accident of the supplementary benefit system.

Until 1983 supplementary benefit paid board and lodgings on one locally determined limit for all types of accommodation. Locally determined maximum limits for private residential care were introduced in November 1983 in order to regularise the system, but instead of restricting expenditure it led to an 'open purse' policy. Homes set their fees to correspond with the maximum limit and as a result costs increased enormously (Bartlett & Challis, 1985). Any elderly person with resources less than £3,000 could seek public funding for a placement in private care without any requirement to demonstrate need.

The three tier system (board and lodgings, residential care home and nursing home limits) along with local limits were scrapped in April 1985 and maximum limits set by central government relating to particular client groups were introduced. However, expenditure has continued to increase as a result of 'the hasty and inadequate policy making' (Bartlett and Challis, 1985). Table 1.4 shows expenditure figures based on a study by Ernst & Whinney (1986).

TABLE 1.4
EXPENDITURE ON SUPPLEMENTARY BENEFIT PAYMENTS FOR PRIVATE HOME RESIDENTS (ENGLAND AND WALES)

Year	Number of claimants	Annual spending	Average payment per week
1978	7,000	6m	£15.7
1984	42,500	190m	£88.0
1986	90,000	460m	£98.0

Expenditure continued to rise with an increasing number of people claiming supplementary benefit. Bradshaw & Gibbs (1987b) estimate that more than 54 per cent of the elderly residents in private and voluntary residential homes are supported in this way. This figure has increased substantially since 1986 when it was estimated that 36 per cent relied on supplementary benefit. (Ernst & Whinney, 1986).

Expenditure not only increased because of greater numbers of elderly people seeking financial support to enter private residential care: part of the increase was due to the fact the market was sensitive to the DHSS limit and as a result charges for homes increased greater than the national limit (Laing & Buisson, 1985). The maximum limit was often taken as the minimum fee by the home owner and as a result residents had to find other means of 'topping up'.

There have been several other financial implications of the availability of supplementary benefit and the expansion of private homes. Many local authorities seized the opportunity to cease offering sponsorship of people needing residential care in the private sector, confident that the supplementary benefit system would pay instead (Peaker, 1986). Sponsorship was also withdrawn from existing residents so that more people were dependent on supplementary benefit. Peaker argues that this has led to a crisis in funding. Insufficient levels of funding for residents with additional disabilities have not only had severe consequences for those residents unable to 'top up' the DHSS level. The initial enthusiasm about available money also brought many couples into buying homes without sufficient capital or understanding of the work (Davidson, 1983). As a result a number have closed after short periods of time, rendering the market unstable. Such instability has been used as an argument against the private provision of residential care.

Political arguments

Several political arguments have been put forward in support of an increasing private market. The political belief in a mixed economy has been enthusiastically promoted by the Conservative government. In relation to the increasing numbers of elderly people there are ongoing fears that the public sector alone cannot cope. In response, the government has made an explicit commitment to 'a mixed economy of welfare' highlighted in documents such as *The way forward* (DHSS, 1977) and *Growing older* (DHSS, 1981a) which encourage alternative sectors to become involved in providing care.

Although the government believes in a mixed economy the current underlying ideology of welfare pluralism is, however, anti-state. This has been demonstrated in reality by the promotion of one sector of welfare - the private sector.

Political arguments in favour of privatisation have focused on the role of the state. The confidence in state welfare, which supposedly existed in the 1950's & 1960's has given way to disillusionment from all sides of the political divide. Some writers such as Webb (1985) and Room (1979) believe there is a good case for a radical reduction in the role of the state and base this on two related perspectives - political and economic liberalism.

The welfare state is seen as unjust, inequitable, failing to redistribute resources (Le Grand, 1982) and promoting social conflict; harbouring abuse and is paternalistic as well as ignorant of the preferences of consumers (Seldon, 1981). Against this background of disillusionment writers of the centre (Judge, Smith & Taylor-Gooby, 1983; Weale, 1983) argue for a greater role for the market as 'an antidote to the development of monolithic state power' (Papadakis & Taylor-Gooby, 1987, p.28). Instead of concentrating on the advantages and disadvantages of non-statutory. provision, there is a pervading belief in the literature quoted above that anything the public sector can do the private sector can do better (Golding, 1983; Leat, 1986). An example of this is the notion of dependency. Privatised provision is assumed not to create dependence (Le Grand & Robinson, 1984; Leat, 1986) unlike the state which has fostered a 'dependency culture'. Walker 1988 in a recent article, however, argues that similar dependencies can be levelled against the private sector. He argues that private entrepreneurs are encouraged to be dependent on the state through the availability of supplementary benefits given to elderly people to enter the private sector:

> That the government places so much importance on encouraging private welfare provision, suggests that it is not dependency as such that it objects to but dependency on the public sector. (Walker, 1988, p.17)

Papadakis & Taylor-Gooby argue, however, that taken individually 'the various arguments about the weakness of state welfare do not add up to a knock down case' (Papadakis & Taylor-Gooby 1987, p.29).

Such debate has put state welfare on the defensive. The most fundamental defence of state production was the assertion of Titmuss (1958) that welfare goods and services were not 'economic goods' because they involved high levels of uncertainty, of risk and of vulnerability on the part of the consumer. This is a weak argument, however, because it accepts the economist's tenets as a starting point. There are a number of practical issues raised in the shift away from the state which are important to the consumer. Not only do the most vulnerable groups suffer but there is a lack of control over the type of provision funded and a difficulty in safeguarding consumer rights.

A favourite left wing argument (for example, Phillips, Vincent & Blacksell, 1988) in defence of the state system hinges around the assumption that 'welfare' cannot survive in the market place partly because of the inherent contradiction between the pursuit of profit and the pursuit of care. Weaver et al (1985a), however, in a study in Norfolk, found that these are compatible and the production of both can be achieved if homes 'balance' the production of profit and care in the right combination. The pursuit of profit is not always at the expense of care as Weaver (1985a) demonstrated. The private sector has to provide a level of care acceptable as a 'commodity' as well as at a 'profitable level'.

Others take such arguments further by claiming that the private sector does not fulfil the same function as the state sector. Phillips, Vincent & Blacksell (1988) again argue that private homes provide a housing function rather than a health or social service function since unlike local authority homes they are not part of a system of sustaining people in their own homes. Because of the different functions served by both sectors, it has been argued that the two sectors provide for very different groups of people; home owners select the 'best', 'low dependency' resident, leaving the more 'needy' vulnerable and 'high' dependency residents to local authority provision. Many critics make the links between these two arguments and assume that private residential care is for 'independent' people who view private homes as an alternate housing function. There is little research evidence, available, however, to support any of these arguments.

There is also no reason to see why private homes cannot extend their function providing day care and short term care similar to that provided by the local authority for the surrounding community. No hard evidence can be found of the private sector only selecting those less dependent. The argument that the private sector fulfils a different function for a different group of people, however, is also weak and has no empirical basis but has continued to be used as a vociferous argument against the expansion of private residential care.

The arguments against privatisation have been well documented (Le Grand & Robinson, 1984), yet most of the claims both for and against have been based on extreme 'ideal' types - a perfect private market versus a perfect form of state provision. An example of such party politicking can be clearly seen in the Labour Party Statement quoted in *The Guardian* (6.2.88) describing privatisation as 'the doctrine of callous individualism'.

Day & Klein (1987), argue that both extreme right and left wing views are nonsense, while Weaver et al (1985b) in their research challenge both sides of the argument:

> It has been demonstrated that the freedom of the market place, untrammelled by state intervention, does not necessarily produce a flowering of secure, home-like communities, where old people can achieve continuity with their existing lives and bold entrepreneurs can reap their just rewards. Yet neither does this support those critics of the left who argue that welfare cannot survive in the market place. Private care is not primarily about greedy small businesses exploiting vulnerable elderly people. Home owners in general show a serious commitment to the business of care. (Weaver 1985b, p.151)

In contrast to the rhetorical arguments, very few empirical studies have been concerned with looking at the consumers view on privatization and the role of the state. Midwinter (1986) however, goes some way to redress this balance in his study revealing that elderly people prefer private domiciliary care because of the flexible character of private services, and the degree of direct control they feel in the relationship between employer and employee.

Arguments in favour of the privatisation of welfare also hinge around the theme of liberty. A counter argument to state paternalism is that the private sector through the operation of market principles gives consumers greater freedom (Seldon, 1981). A justification for increasing the mixed economy of welfare has been that it increases choice. Ray Whitney stated:

> A mix, which implies individual choice, freedom and responsibility is what most people welcome. (Whitney quoted in House of Commons, 1986, col. 1136)

One assumption on which the argument for choice hinges is that considerable sections of the elderly population are affluent, particularly through home ownership and occupational pensions (Bessell, 1983a; Thatcher, 1962; Moore, 1988), and therefore have the opportunity to choose between alternative sectors of care. As a result of their increasing purchasing power they would argue that elderly people have also changed their attitude toward private welfare. Midwinter writes:

> Old peoples' perceptions of need seem to have changed, so that they expect more care and help and are less likely to struggle on when they see it is available at reasonable cost. (Midwinter1986, p.4)

However, the idea that the increase in the numbers of private homes increases choice is something of a myth (Higgins, 1985). The appeal of 'choice' is not sufficient to guarantee that the interests of the elderly will be met (Phillips, Vincent & Blacksell, 1988). The empirically based literature on admissions to private residential care, captures a recurring issue - the lack of choice at every stage in the process (Challis, 1985; Weaver, 1985b) - from the point at which admission to care is considered (when decisions are taken by relatives), through the assessment of 'need for care' (defined by professionals) to the decision to enter (often Hobson's choice).

Freedom of choice also hinges on several conditions, which in regard to elderly people entering care are questionable. Writers such as Bessell (1983a) fail to acknowledge that only a minority of elderly people who are in need of care have the ability or opportunity to choose between a variety of options. The choice to remain at home or enter a residential home depends on the availability of community care resources - yet if local authorities spending is too high in this area they are penalized and lose their grant from central government. Such a contradiction or 'perverse incentive' should be redressed so that private residential care can be part of a range of options and not inevitable.

Similarly contradictions exist in the choice between private homes. Market principles of supply and demand require 'perfect knowledge' yet many elderly people lack the information on which to base a decision (Vincent, Tibbenham & Phillips, 1987). Some knowledge can only be acquired after entry but the ability of residents (particularly those with disabilities) to pick and choose between one home or another is restricted as they cannot exercise trial and error choice as a purchaser of market goods in a supermarket (Vincent & Phillips, 1987). Choice to remain at home or enter residential care is in reality limited to a few people. The kind of person and under what circumstances they can exercise choice, however, has not been recorded in much of the research.

On the basis of existing evidence 'the proportion of residents exercising choice is so small that "consumer choice" serves no regulatory function' (Weaver 1985a & b). Biggs concludes:

> To leave quality of care and participation to market forces is little more than a statement of ideological belief rather than concern for the reality of choice on the part of old people. The possibility of making informed decisions about potential residences is severely restricted. (Biggs 1987b, p.79)

Walker (1988) also illustrates that consumer sovereignty is irrelevant because consumers are manipulated by commercial concerns. There is support also for the argument that the only choice that does exist lies with the proprietor (Biggs, 1987a, p.78). Vincent & Phillips in their study in Devon in 1985 found that the power of home owners in selecting residents together with restrictions because of high fees, particularly to those on supplementary benefit, limited the exercise of choice.

There is, however, evidence to suggest that in a number of cases it is irrelevant whether a public or private placement is followed, because the family just want relief. Vickers & Yarrow (1985) found that consumers could not care less who owned the service they used, particularly in a crisis (Phillips & Vincent, 1986a).

Economic arguments

Parallel to the debates on the political disillusionment of the welfare state are arguments that state welfare impedes economic growth and wealth creation (Minford, 1984). This notion was supported when a Treasury statement in 1979 put the level of public expenditure at the heart of Britain's economic difficulties. Large chunks of such expenditure were going into social service provision for elderly people.

The assumption implied in such statements was that the welfare state should be more cost-effective, efficient, better value for money, and more akin to the private sector (DHSS, 1977; DHSS 1981b; DHSS 1981a; Judge et al, 1983). Although there is some evidence to suggest that private enterprise can be more efficient (Judge & Knapp, 1985) it has been argued that the goal of welfare has become subservient to the goal of economic growth and efficiency (Tinker, 1981; Pinker, 1983; Papadakis & Taylor- Gooby, 1987). Efficiency and effectiveness of the service, however, depends on the balance of care against need and not just on economic principles (Bosanquet, 1978).

The government's line has been that the private sector promotes wealth which is a necessary precondition for the development of welfare. There is also an underlying assumption, that such wealth will 'trickle down'. In contrast, several studies - Walker & Walker (1987) and The Archbishop of Canterbury's study *'Faith in the city'* (1985) - show that divisions between rich and poor in society have become greater.

Other evidence of efficiency in the private sector is lacking and where there is evidence it shows that the free market is not highly efficient and self adjusting as it does not depend on genuine competition without duplication: 'The market is fragmented and compartmentalised with individual budgets and systems operating different rules' (Maynard, 1987).

In total, however, the evidence is not overwhelming or conclusive one way or the other. There is little basis on which to say one sector is more efficient or effective, than the other, or even better or worse than the other, if one assesses all the political, ethical and economic arguments together.

The expression of social concern

Arguments advanced by protagonists of private care focus on the belief that quality of care is better in the private sector. Market principles, they assume, ensure that the proprietors who provide inadequate standards of care will be weeded out of the market.

Recent documentary evidence (*The Granny Business*, ITV 1987; NUPE, 1986) emotionally demonstrates however, that the private sector is no better than the local authority sector in promoting 'adequate' standards of care, and that market principles do not ensure 'bogus' or 'cowboy' operators 'attracted by potentially high profits with no desire to care for old people' (NUPE, 1986, p.16) are driven out of the market.

The major social concern has focused on standards of care and particularly the abuse of elderly people. Early warnings based on the American experience and illustrated by Vladeck (1980) went unheeded with examples of similar psychological and physical abuse found across this country.

Newspaper headlines reporting 'The mistress at home is banned' (*Eastern Evening News*, 24.5.87); 'Wide abuse in private homes for the elderly - care code flouted by profiteers' (Hoyland, 1986) and 'Granny farm homes for the old' (*Daily Telegraph*, 30.10.86) conjure up the often distorted sensationalist view of the private sector.

The NUPE report '*The realities of home life*' (1986) graphically illustrates case studies of abuse found in private homes which centre around overcrowding, poor food, dangerous medical practices, inhuman treatment, inadequate fire standards, regimentation, understaffing, low pay and atrocious working conditions.

Another bleak portrait of life in one part of the private sector was broadcast revealing a story of neglect, filth, and indignity in private homes in Kent. One newspaper reported the following day: 'Elderly people are forgotten ones, left to rot' (*Guardian*, 8.10.87). Not only does the media generalise the situation in the private sector, government opponents also make sweeping statements about 'handsome profits being made at the expense of the old' (House of Commons, 1986, col. 1135).

An expression of concern in private sector developments has stemmed not only from worries about elderly people being exploited in a private market but has come as a consequence of the heavy critique of institutional care in the 1970's. Anyone could be forgiven for assuming such literature referred to the situation in public institutions of the early 1970's.

Less than a handful of studies, however, turn to the benefits which residents may experience from living in a private home. In reality the horrors of residential life outlined by Meacher (1972) and others have not been replicated on such a wide scale. Although the popular press have taken one or two examples of bad practice, what such observers of the private sector fail to see is the way the private sector has accommodated the changing nature of need. Over and above the basic 'welfare' provision of tending, food, supply of daily care and so on, residents demand privacy, independence and comfort in a pleasant homely setting. The private sector attempts to accommodate such demand.

Although several commentators condemn the private system, (for example, Ackland, 1987) there is nothing to say that public care is superior. A cautious reminder to local authority advocates and those castigating the private sector as 'exploitative and bad' is the recent evidence of 'scandalous abuse' found in local authority homes in Southwark and Camden (Clough, 1987).

More detailed research on abuse in the private sector is lacking, possibly because widespread abuse doesn't abound. Reports, quoted above, however, demonstrate that in terms of quality of care, both sectors vary and 'just as the private sector has no monopoly on scandals, so the private sector has no monopoly on excellence' (Day, 1985, p.285).

The concern about abuse, however, has had some positive side effects with the development of a new code of practice: *Home Life* (Avebury, 1984) being drawn up following the Registered Homes Act 1980 and subsequent legislation in the form of the Registered Homes Act, 1984.

Registration. The main purpose of the registration legislation is to raise the standard of care and prevent the exploitation of frail and vulnerable people (Challis, 1985). This presupposes that until people's expectations change and they become more aware of the variations in standards, the 'magic of market forces alone will not generate quality control' (Grindod, Leigh, Smith, 1987, p.18; BASW, 1986). In the current situation it is argued that only sensitive but uncompromising enforcement of the legislation will avoid the worst excesses of commercially-based care (Johnson, 1983 and 1984; Murray, 1984).

Can the legislation achieve its objectives?

Evidence points to the fact that the legislation is having a variable impact. Although the Registered Homes Act 1984 reinforced the framework of accountability set up through previous legislation, the interpretation and enforcement of this act was, and still is left to the registering authority (Brooke-Ross, 1986a). As a result, there have been varying standards across the country (DHSS, 1987a) and 'striking differences' have been found in standards, staffing, procedures and guidance (Kellaher et al, 1988).

The legislation also has a limited effect in providing high care standards because of the difficulties in defining 'the minimum level of care' (Bartlett & Brooke-Ross, 1986). The elements in defining levels of care, around issues such as individuality and autonomy are not always accessible and amenable to a high degree of routine treatment and will, therefore, vary depending on who defines good and bad care. Examples of such varying definitions can be found in the evidence presented to tribunals in the last few years, which demonstrates that the criteria on which the registering authority and the appeal judge regard as good or bad practice may differ (Carson, 1985).

Cassam notes that 20 per cent of cases (out of a sample of 46) in tribunals were upheld with private proprietors continuing in business. He concludes that 'it is unlikely that poor practice as distinct from bad practice can really be rooted out by legal action' (Cassam, 1987a, p.12).

Good practice covering aspects of choice and autonomy are also difficult to enforce because of the voluntary nature of the code of practice: *Home life*, (Avebury, 1984).

Others believe that good standards in the private sector can be achieved through adequate support from the registering authority (Jolly, 1986) yet the pressure on staff caused by the exponential growth in numbers of private homes makes their supportive role difficult. Challis (1985) also found that the registration officers knowledge and understanding of the complex processes in the commercial sector were thin.

Recent empirical evidence, however, calls for greater optimism. Physical standards and practical aspects of care delivery in existing homes have been raised 'by the routinisation of registration and inspection work' (Kellaher et al, 1988, p.122; BASW, 1986; Brooke-Ross, 1986b). There has also been a move to self-regulation in an attempt to improve standards and to set minimum standards for new proprietors. Home Owners Associations - locally and nationally - dissatisfied with existing registration arrangements have co-operated and attempted to consolidate their position through a control system by the move toward an independent national inspectorate (Beddoe, 1985b). Many social service departments, however, view this with scepticism, expressing their view that the assessment of quality of care cannot be replaced by an association which claims to know a good commercial enterprise when they see one.

The ineffectiveness of legislation to identify and respond to abuse leads some writers such as Brooke-Ross to comment that the only:

> Real way to raise standards and improve the intangible aspects of quality control cannot be through enforcement but by counselling, the development role and the partnership between public, private and voluntary sectors. (Brooke-Ross, 1986b, p.15)

Regulation does appear to work well in authorities who:

> Are coming to terms with private care and can accommodate to the world of welfare pluralism - irrespective of an authority's location on a political spectrum. (Kellaher et al, 1988, p.121)

The Norfolk model is upheld as a practical example of effective 'partnership and professional interaction between the two sectors', and is based on the assumption that problems involving styles and principles of care are resolvable by rational enquiry and debate (Norfolk County Council, 1985). Although this is seen as 'a fruitful way forward' (Cassam, 1987, p.67) balancing regulation and partnership is 'like walking a tightrope'. Some would argue further that the talk of partnership is just rhetoric divorced from practice (Kellaher et al, 1988).

The Centre for Environmental and Social Studies in Ageing (CESSA) study stated:

> Senior managers in 42 authorities found partnership a difficult concept to address, particularly as the relationship was unequal. (Kellaher et al, 1988, p.118)

Members of the private sector also view the relationship as one sided and find the dual role of policing and friendship a confusing and conflicting one (Beddoe, 1988). It is therefore not easy to find common ground between the two sectors apart from their concern for the well-being of old people in care.

The discussion around 'common interests' (not yet seen in the literature), appears increasingly necessary because the private sector needs to avoid the mistakes of the public sector and to develop as part of an integrated local plan for residential care. This will be increasingly difficult under present circumstances as the growth of private residential care is contradictory to the policy of keeping people at home and even if community care is advocated by this sector, private homes may lack the necessary relationships with local support networks to encourage rehabilitation (Etherington, 1984; McCoy, 1984).

Although necessary, there are other inherent difficulties. The non-statutory sector is not a single entity or a 'partnership' within itself; it holds very different views about its development and relationship with the statutory sector. It will need to change its hostile view of this relationship where it sees itself 'restricted by red tape' (Churchill, 1985) and subject to

'Gestapo tactics' (Parsons, 1986) if it is to develop a common strategy for elderly people. Alongside this, the public sector will 'need to think with clarity, speak with truth and act with honesty, if they want the partnership to work' (Clarke, 1985). Further work on the nature of private sector provision is therefore necessary and timely.

The most important partnership, however, is with consumers (Biggs, 1987a), and not just consumers of the private sector but of the public sector. This section has shown that a close eye is being kept on the private sector, because of the possible repetition of abuse found in the early 1970's in the public sector. Yet regulation has not been equally applied to the public sector. Also, although the well being of residents is sometimes put forward as an argument by proprietors of registration authorities, 'in legislation they are the silent third party' (Brooke-Ross, 1987, p.13).

Social work and the private sector

Social workers concerned with the needs of individual clients are placed in a key 'boundary' position between public and private welfare systems. Because social workers are naturally seen as professional advocates and key people in the process of admission, there is a case to be made for the development of 'partnership' to take place between the sectors at this practice based level. It could also be argued from the literature that the growth of private residential care, however, demands a change in the role for social workers particularly when their 'traditional' role is taken by relatives.

Social work practice literature such as BASW 1984, assumes the need for social workers to work within the private sector.

> Insofar as social workers are concerned with the care of vulnerable old people they will increasingly have to concern themselves with non-state forms of provision. (Challis, 1985, p.44)

There are several areas, such as admission, in which it would seem appropriate that the social worker transfer skills developed within the public arena of welfare. These may also be supplemented by new roles such as involvement in the process of registration.

The Social Services Inspectorate (DHSS, 1987a), reporting on the 'Impact of the Registered Homes Act 1984' stated:

> Inspection work needs to be characterised by a high degree of professional content and occasionally needs supporting by an input from staff with specialist expertise in the relevant field of care'. (DHSS, 1987a p.16)

Registration and inspection should, therefore, not be seen as an administrative task but one requiring the professional skills of a social worker in exercising judgement about homes, their owners and quality of care. Social workers working with individual clients are well placed to detect unregistered and questionable provision (Challis, 1985) and can ensure there is an acceptable minimum for all (Bessell, 1983b).

Another major potential area of involvement for social workers in the private sector is in assessing the elderly people's need for care. The present system of supplementary benefit allows fees to be paid on an individual financial basis regardless of whether the person needs care. Without assessment there is a fear that people enter care unnecessarily and inappropriately while wasting scarce public resources (*The Times* 10.5.88). Recent evidence (Bradshaw & Gibbs, 1988) contradicts this and reports that the proportion of elderly people in private and voluntary homes in four pilot study areas found not to be in need of care was very small.

Assessment can play a vital role and involve the social worker in assessing the person's needs and wishes independently of any other decisions therefore acting in the best interests of the client.

Similarly other important areas for the social worker in the private sector can be highlighted from the literature relating to their role in the public sector. For example, it is crucial to ensure the right care is arranged, and there is continued contact with the client once in residential care.

The social worker can also give clients an informed choice - in terms of the range of possible packages of care and information on private and local authority homes. The British Association of Social Workers (BASW) reinforces the social workers role in their guidelines:

> Holding the balance in complex social situations is a task which requires distinctive social work skills ... it requires a social worker who will pay primary regard to the fundamental principles of residential care. (BASW 1984, p.9)

This statement, it appears, fails to acknowledge the position in which social workers as public sector agents find themselves - it assumes they feel comfortable working within an alternative system based on competition and ability to pay.

Attitudes of the social work profession to the private sector. The debate about the involvement of social workers in the private sector has become 'burdened by political and professional dogmatism on all sides' (Bessell, 1983b, p.14).

Many social workers on the left regard any involvement in private residential care as promoting an unacceptable form of welfare and state their position as 'non-cooperation' (Benson, 1987, p.21). Not only are social workers concerned about:

> The increasing volume of work resulting from increasing numbers requesting assistance but they express an uncomfortable feeling about colluding with relatives wishing to use the private sector. (Hemsley, 1985, p.15)

In some cases they portray open hostility (Bradshaw & Gibbs, 1987a). Many social workers, however, are hypocritical in levelling their criticism against private care. Literature on the relationship between the social worker and the public sector reveals that equity and fairness do not operate in the sector where they have a degree of control because of the different swop systems and bureaucratic wranglings.

The cautious stance which many social workers take in 'recommending' the 'exploitative' private sector reflects their own position. As public agency representatives, some are worried that private sector growth devalues their own role and removes incentives from the local authority to improve the situation. From a personal point of view, many are worried about their vulnerable position in the firing line of relatives or residents if anything goes wrong with the placement (BASW, 1984 and 1986). Transferring skills from one sector to another, therefore, may not be as straightforward as much of the practice based literature assumes.

Despite overall ambiguity in role and attitude, very few authorities have issued guidelines on how to proceed in effectively translating the notion of partnership into practice at a fieldwork level. This may leave social workers making their own decisions about their level of involvement, although there is no current research on this aspect of practice.

The lack of trust and suspicion is not just one way. Some former private sector proprietors view social workers 'non cooperative stance as 'blinkered, arrogant and a reflection of self interest' (Beddoe, 1985a, p.15). Private sector operators dislike social work interference, particularly in the area of assessment for need of care. They feel it is wrong to put the 'consumer in the passenger seat with the professional in the driving seat' (Beddoe, 1988).

In terms of monitoring the level and content of continuing social work involvement in the private sector, there is a noticeable absence of research. The attractiveness of the private sector to social work in terms of its flexibility and freedom from bureaucratic hurdles has not been documented.

The marginalisation of social work. Several studies reveal that social workers do not become involved in all admissions to private residential care (Willcocks et al, 1987; Phillips, Vincent & Blacksell, 1988), even for those elderly people in need of residential care (Bradshaw & Gibbs, 1988). There is little evidence to say whether this is due to their political opposition, or whether they are ignored by other professionals and relatives. However, the studies reveal that relatives are the main operators in the process of admission (The Association of Directors of Social Services, 1985; BASW 1984; Weaver 1985a&b; Bartlett & Challis (undated)).

The marginal position of the social worker is interesting in light of the current debate on social work assessment of potential private sector residents. Despite the welcomed response to the Firth Report's (DHSS, 1987b) suggestion of a proper assessment for entry to private residential care, it is presumed that the task of assessment will fall on social workers. This places a burden on them to become gatekeepers to both cash and care. Although, as Gibbs & Bradshaw (1988, p.591) state 'there is no intrinsic barrier to employing social workers to assess elderly person's needs for residential care in the independent sector' introducing public gatekeeping into the private sector distorts the market (Kay, 1987) and gives the local authority unfair advantage over the private sector inconsistent with the mixed economy of welfare (Gibbs & Bradshaw, 1987).

Some private home owners see such public sector intrusion as dangerously prone to political partiality, bureaucracy and even corruption and find it unacceptable (Mabon, 1989).

The differences between the sectors are important to consider in respect of assessment for entry. The assessment skills and procedures used for local authority accommodation (where allocation is heavily influenced by the admission criteria set by individual homes or by the 'urgency' of the admission) are not readily transferable to the private sector and new kinds of assessment capable of judging the need for residential care, quite separately from decisions about entry to particular homes will be necessary.

Evidence from Wilkin & Jolly (1979) shows that social workers often inappropriately place people in the 'wrong' care settings and this has major implications for placing people in a sector about which social workers hold less information.

If public sector assessment of private sector applicants applying for supplementary benefit were to come about then the literature would show far reaching implications for the social work role. If one of Firth's (DHSS, 1987b) recommendations of the Local Authority taking responsibility for all residential provision is taken on board, then social workers will move from a marginal position to one of power and significance in the allocation of elderly people to private and public residential homes.

Conclusion

This literature review has attempted to demonstrate the changing nature of welfare for elderly people in the late twentieth century. In so doing, it raises a whole gamut of issues, including the attitude of society towards elderly people. There has been an ageist attitude inherent in policy development. Older people have been viewed in a negative light, not only because of their increasing numbers but working with older people was often seen as depressing and worthless by the social work profession. A spin off of the growth of the private sector has been that elderly people have increased their potential in the eyes of society as potential consumers in the market place. This has given them a voice. The effects of political ideologies, statistical evidence of demographic trends and the increasing emphasis of private residential care rather than state provision have been raised as issues.

Several themes, however, recur:

1. Despite the vociferous critique of institutional life in the 1960's and its subsequent ad hoc development, and being viewed as 'the last resort' residential care has remained a dominant form of provision for elderly people. The change is that residential care is no longer solely provided by the state but increasingly by the private sector.

2. The burgeoning of the private sector is not only a response to increasing numbers of frail elderly people or to the decreasing number of care-givers in the family, but a result of the government's promotion of private welfare through the supplementary benefit system. One body of literature argues that such 'commodification' of welfare has enabled elderly people to exercise choice over their future direction of care. Other literature views the private market as exploitative and profit-making with little concern for vulnerable elderly people. Such reactions to private sector influence, however, tend to

occur almost regardless of the specific issue. Furthermore, they seem to be based upon the supposition that the alternatives are state provision or private enterprise, forgetting that the state may subsidize or regulate the private market. Such regulation, however, places the state in a contradictory relationship with the private sector, because not only does it 'police' the private residential sector, but its agents (ie. registration officers) are engaged in a move toward a partnership between the two sectors.

This dual role presents difficulties for those working on the boundary between the two sectors, particularly for social workers who may be professionally and personally opposed to private care. The literature highlights the confusion over the social workers role in the public sector but has little to say about the nature of social work in the private sector.

3. It is not only the formal sectors of welfare that shoulder the responsibility of increasing numbers of frail elderly people. The stress throughout this literature review has been on the importance of the family in its care for elderly relatives. The literature highlights the often contradictory relationship between family and state but no literature source has addressed the issue of the relationship between the family and the private sector.

This review also has shown the extent to which elderly people are neglected in the development of welfare provision. How best to provide care for an individual based on their preference has taken a back seat in discussion to how such care can be provided most economically. Although there is nothing intrinsically wrong in this, the assumption that this is the only way forward must be questioned if economic efficiency and social equality are to be sought as guiding principles.

2 Methodology

Research design

The investigation into 'the process of admission into private residential care for elderly people' was funded from September 1985 to September 1987 by the Economic and Social Research Council and involved collaboration between the University of East Anglia and Suffolk Social Services Department.

The timing of this study was opportune with the expansion of private provision in the county of Suffolk and with the increasing need to incorporate the private sector in both planning residential provision and policy making in the future. Apart from basic numerical data, little was known about residents in private residential homes in the United Kingdom, why and how they came into a private rather than a local authority home.

The main aim of the study was to look at the critical steps in the pathways and processes operating in the admission of elderly people into private residential care: that is, to explore the ways in which people became residents, why they became residents, what choices were available and what help they received during the process of admission.

The investigation consisted of a main study involving interviews with 200 residents in a representative sample of 39 private residential homes in the county of Suffolk. Interviews with elderly people, their relatives and professionals in the process were conducted during a six month period from April to September 1986. The contract with Suffolk Social Services Department necessitated a focus on the private sector but to reach a useful conclusion it was recognised that comparative data was needed. As a result, the study incorporated data from the public sector which was used in a secondary fashion for comparative purposes only. This second stage of interviews with local authority residents took place between March and September 1987.

This chapter describes the methods of data collection, sampling procedures and methods used in interviewing which were tested in the field in a pilot study and used in the main investigation. The conclusion looks at the problems of carrying out this kind of research and outlines the limitations of these particular data sets, together with considerations for future research studies of this nature.

The exploratory and pilot studies

An exploratory study was carried out in the first three months with the purpose of clarifying the problem for investigation and attempting a clear understanding of the substance of the topic. Central to this stage was to look at what was feasible from a practical point of view and how efficiently the subject could be investigated in the field. These objectives were explored in three ways:

a) by a review of the literature (Chapter 1);
b) an 'experience study' (Jahoda et al, 1951, p.36) which took the form of discussions with professionals and specialists, both in practice and academic circles reflecting a wide variety of viewpoints;
c) a case study approach - 14 residents in 5 homes in Norfolk were interviewed regarding their pattern of admission, and life prior to and after admission. The main themes were teased out and clarified through the series of interviews. From the content of these exploratory interviews, questionnaires were designed and methods of interviewing investigated.

A content analysis after the exploratory stage defined seven main areas for further investigation.

1. Life of the resident prior to admission

2. The event(s) in the process leading to admission

3. Significant people involved in the process

4. Reflections on the process by the resident

5. Life as it was at the point of admission

6. Life as it is now

7. Financial circumstances relevant to the admission process

The seven areas identified acted as a framework for the pilot study and were included in the design of the interview schedules. In order to check the viability of the research strategy and the suitability of the various methods of data collection proposed, a pilot study was designed to incorporate the central features of the main consumer study.

The pilot study took place between January and March 1986 in two areas of Suffolk (Babergh and Western) not chosen for the main study in order to keep the areas 'clean' for the main research. Three homes were randomly selected for the pilot, including 15 residents, 8 relatives and 6 professionals who were interviewed in depth.

The pilot study was carried out specifically to test the viability and practical feasibility of using several interview schedules and techniques, a sampling framework and access to residents. The organisation of the fieldwork and collection and reporting of data were also evaluated at this stage.

This stage confirmed the importance of a semi-directive approach with the interview checklists and questionnaires and as the pilot study progressed, it became clear that the two main approaches employed - an unstructured schedule and a checklist - were both necessary to obtain the range of information.

The main themes that emerged from the pilot study in need of further clarification were:

1. Who makes up the population of private residential homes?

2. By what route do they gain admission?

3. Who were the significant operators in the process?

4. Were viable alternatives available?

5. Were elderly people influential and able to exercise choice in the process? If so, were they a particular kind of resident?

On completion of the pilot study, an interim report was prepared and circulated to the eight home owners for discussion and feedback. The report highlighted the decision-making process of home owners, the levels of satisfaction expressed by residents and relatives and the sometimes tricky relationship between social workers and the private sector. This report was also discussed with the Director of Social Services and other professionals in social work and related research fields. Their comments, gratefully received, were influential in the amendments made in planning the main study and in the continual development of ideas.

Local authority pilot study

A pilot study was carried out in two local authority homes outside the main study area in January 1987. Few amendments were made.

The main study: the Suffolk context

The following pages introduce the study by looking at how the Suffolk sample was selected; the different methods used in interviewing; the success of access and the response rate; the frameworks used for recording, coding and analysing the data and, finally, the reliability and validity of the measures used, along with the limitations of the data collected.

The increasing numbers of elderly people nationally are reflected in the growth of the elderly population in Suffolk. Between 1981 and 1988 the number of people aged over 75 years has risen by about twenty per cent - from 38,479 to an estimated 46,329. By 1996, if growth continues there will be an increase in demand to 52,565 elderly people aged 75 years and over, indicating a thirty-seven per cent growth since 1981 (Suffolk County Council, 1986b).

In comparison with national figures (see Chapter One) the percentage of those aged 75 and above will be higher in this county than the national average (Darton and McCoy, 1981).

Increases in population consequently increases the demand for services. In terms of residential provision, local authority growth has not kept pace with these demographic increases. Between 1971-1980 the local authority increased its residential provision by twenty-five per cent and in the same period the population aged 75 and over rose by twenty-two per cent. Since then, however, the rate of public sector growth has slowed down and continues to do so. Such depressed growth was mainly due to two factors - the slow time lag inevitable in buildings of new provision coming on stream and the closing down in the 1970s of the old workhouse type of provision (McCoy, 1985).

At the same time as the slowing down, the private sector has steadily grown. The bulk of this growth in Suffolk has been since 1980. By 1984 the number of beds registered in the public and private sectors was equal in all areas. By 1988 the private and voluntary sectors (2,000) had overtaken the local authority sector (1,500; figures based on Suffolk's residential accommodation returned to Department of Health 1988, DoH 1989).

The private sector has filled the gap in residential provision and has done so by providing a similar provision. The two sectors in 1980 were found to have residents of similar age, need for care and degree of disability (McKenzie and Baldock, 1981).

This independent research study concluded that because of the similarity (ie. the two sectors catered for similarly dependent residents), with deteriorating levels of local authority provision and the increasing need for residential care the private sector could be harnessed as an additional resource (McKenzie and Baldock, 1981).

While there has been some acknowledgement of this growth in policy regarding residential care, Suffolk had until 1986 been slow to include the private sector into its planning mechanism - with the result that there has been a paucity of policy statements and planning objectives including the private sector.

This has, however, reflected two difficulties:

1. Policy adopted by Suffolk has concentrated on the differences between the two sectors - seeing private care offering something different to their provision of residential care as a community resource.

DIAGRAM 2.1
RESIDENTIAL CARE FOR ELDERLY PEOPLE IN SUFFOLK: LOCAL AUTHORITY, PRIVATE AND VOLUNTARY SECTORS COMPARED (1984)

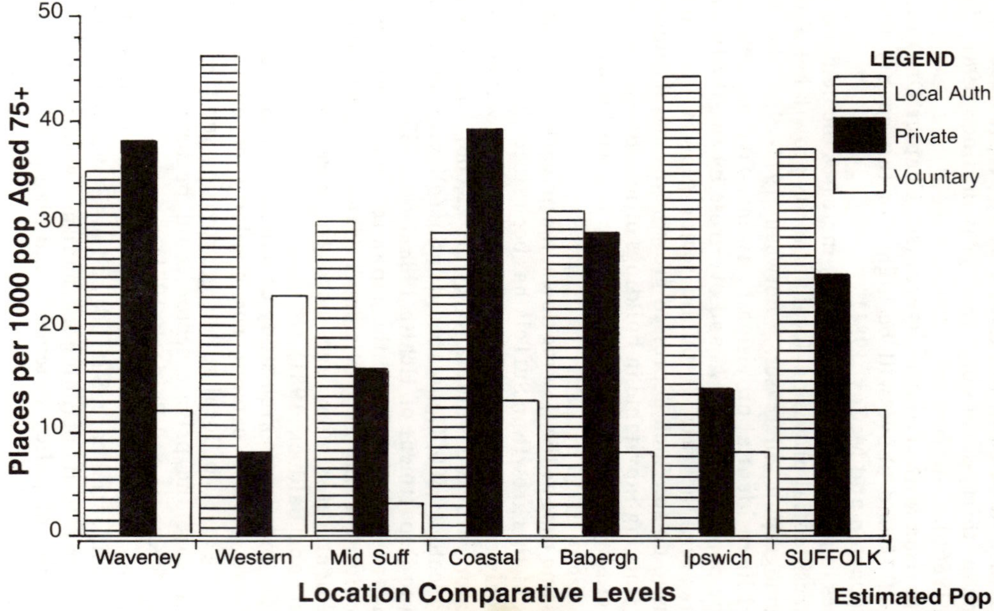

Source: McCoy (1989) 'Privatisation of residential care for elderly people: the data hare and the policy tortoise?', *Research, Policy and Planning*, vol.3(1), p.15

2. Also the growth of the private sector in Suffolk (Diagram 2.1) has not been uniform across the county. Divisions within Suffolk show disparity (Diagrams 2.2 and 2.3). In Ipswich, Mid-Suffolk and Babergh the local authority held most beds, whereas in the divisions of Suffolk Coastal and Waveney (along the coastal belt) the private sector has greater provision than the local authority. This creates difficulty for planning across the county and for county-wide policy to be sensitive to local need.

The geographical differences, however, were used in this study to derive a representative sample from both sectors and from the county as a whole.

Sample selection

Five separate stages of sampling involved sampling areas, residential homes, residents, relatives and professionals.

(a) Geographical areas (Diagram 2.2). In December 1985, there existed 78 private residential homes in Suffolk with a population of 1,240 residents (figures were based on the number of registered places in private homes when at full capacity, obtained from the County Council's list of registered private and voluntary homes for elderly people). Four years later (April 1989), the population had increased to 1,605 persons in ninety private homes. Nevertheless, despite this growth, there is no reason to believe that the research is not applicable.

It was not feasible to include all 78 homes in the study given the possible lengthy negotiation needed to gain access, the time involved in interviewing and the distance to be covered across the County.

Following a review of a number of characteristics, it was decided to stratify the sample on the presence of local authority and private sector homes in the county. The geographical dimension covered all the differences in supply and demand. The four areas chosen were Waveney, Ipswich, Mid-Suffolk and Suffolk Coastal - each area contrasting in its proportion of local authority and private registered homes (Table 2.1). The distribution and proportion of local authority and private registered homes is shown in Diagram 2.3.

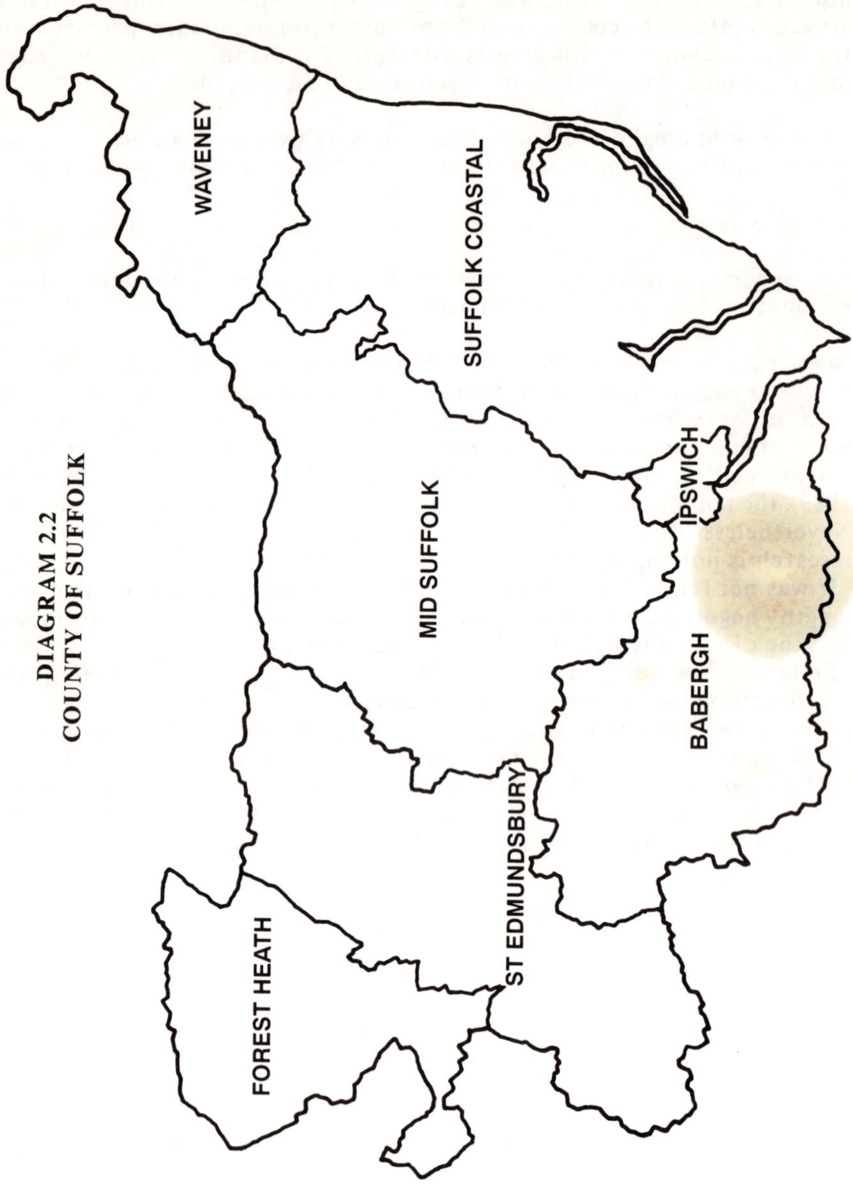

DIAGRAM 2.2
COUNTY OF SUFFOLK

DIAGRAM 2.3
DISTRIBUTION AND PROPORTION OF LOCAL AUTHORITY AND PRIVATE REGISTERED BEDS IN FOUR CHOSEN AREAS OF SUFFOLK (1985)

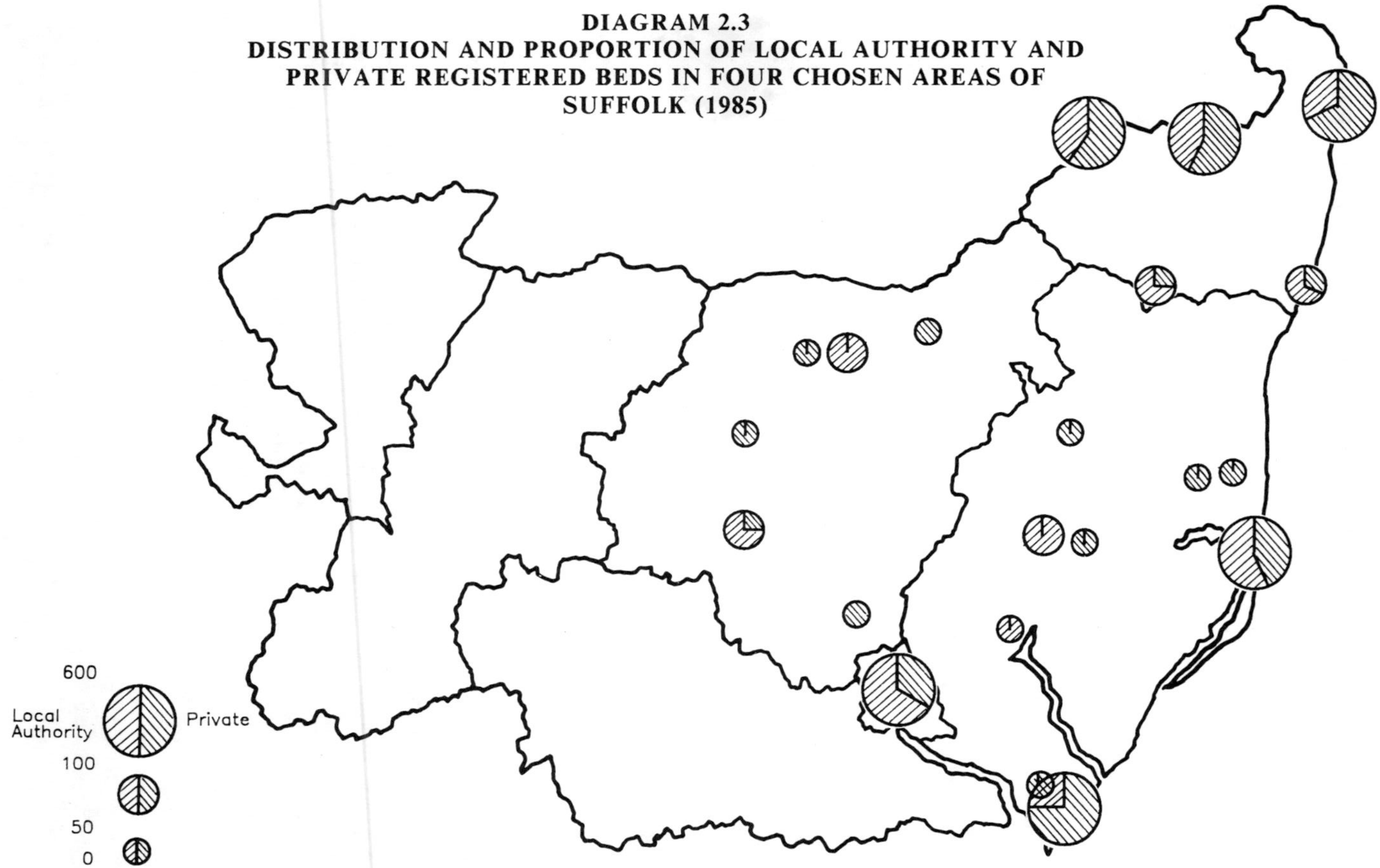

TABLE 2.1
SAMPLE AREAS FOR STUDY (BASED ON 1985 FIGURES)

	local authority residents	private sector residents	no. of private homes	no. of residents in private homes
Waveney	high	high	23	361
Ipswich	high	low	10	174
Mid-Suffolk	low	low	7	93
Suffolk Coastal	low	high	22	370
			62	998

(not included in the main study, but included in the pilot study)

Babergh	low	high
Western	high	low

	number of local authority homes	number of residents in local authority homes
Waveney	6	291
Ipswich	7	360
Mid-Suffolk	3	148
Suffolk Coastal	6	234
	22	1033

(b) Sample of homes. The aim was to select a representative sample of private residential homes in the four areas chosen. The sample was to be statistically representative and also manageable in practical terms of size and travel distance between the homes.

Initially, it was planned to cover all homes in the four areas based on the fact that three residents per home would be interviewed. However, the average number of new residents proved to be six per home and individual homes were, therefore, selected randomly in each of the four areas with the use of a random numbers table (White, Yeates & Skipworth, 1974). The total number of homes per area were not weighted according to whether they had high or low private provision in relation to public provision. Only thirty-nine homes were contacted before the target figure of two hundred residents was reached.

TABLE 2.2
NUMBER OF HOMES COVERED IN EACH AREA

	private	local authority	all
Waveney	13	5	18
Ipswich	6	5	11
Mid-Suffolk	6	2	8
Suffolk Coastal	14	4	18
	39 (63%)	16 (73%)	55

A list of local authority homes was obtained and a random sample was taken following the same procedure as the selection in the private sector. It is believed that the sample of homes obtained was satisfactorily representative of homes in Suffolk. However, no claims can be made in terms of its representiveness of homes in England and the United Kingdom as a whole.

(c) Samples of residents. A crucial element in the design of this study was the selection of residents which would reflect the range of different background circumstances and pathways into residential care.

Residents who entered private residential homes within the period of a year prior to the interview were selected for three reasons:

a) to keep the sample numbers manageable in practical terms;

b) because the memory of the elderly person in respect of life prior to admission and their experience of the process may fade with time, particularly if a year or more has lapsed;

c) at the time of interview, professionals and relatives were more likely to be in the same location as at the time of admission, thus facilitating contact and access.

To arrive at the figure of 200, the total population of new residents in each home (that is, those who arrived in each home immediately one year prior to the study) were interviewed. Both permanent (181) and short-stay residents (19) were interviewed, irrespective of dependency or level of confusion.

(d) The local authority sample of residents. A target figure of 120 residents was chosen for the local authority study and the numbers of residents admitted within the year were obtained for the four areas from '*Residential and Day Care Services for Elderly People*' (Suffolk Social Services Department, 1986a).

A target population for each area was calculated by:

$$\frac{\text{number of new entrants in 1 area}}{\text{number of new entrants in 4 areas}} \times 120$$

The sampling procedure for residents differed slightly in this second stage because local authority homes admitted more residents in the previous year than were required for the sample. [In contrast, the 200 people interviewed in the private sector represented 90 per cent of the residents admitted within the year to the private sector in the areas chosen.] The target population per local authority home was therefore calculated:

$$\frac{\text{number of residents admitted to each home}}{\text{number of residents admitted in the particular area}} \times \text{target population for the area}$$

A random sample of new residents was then taken within each home (homes were again selected through a random sample).

(e) A sample of relatives and professionals. To add depth to the study, two additional sets of interviews were undertaken, one with relatives and the other with professionals 'significantly' involved in the process of each individual resident's admission into care. This not only provided an additional perspective to the process but gave a reliability check on the accounts of residents.

Allowing for one relative and one professional interview per resident, the potential number of interviews in the private sector study reached 600.

Relatives and professionals were selected in the local authority study on an identical basis. Because admission to a local authority home required a social worker to assess the need for residential care, all 120 social workers were identified as the significant professional. The potential number of interviews in the local authority study therefore was 360.

Methods of interviewing

(1) Residents. The main source of information concerning the process of admission came from the new residents themselves and for this reason the design of the residents' questionnaire was regarded as a focal point of the study.

A structured questionnaire aimed at getting 'common' data in order to construct a profile of the new resident. This included information related to age, marital status, gender, physical and mental state. A background picture was also assembled concerning the person's situation prior to admission, including location and type of accommodation, household composition and support at home, both formal and informal. This provided the vital framework for the movements that led to private residential care.

The interview discussion centred around life circumstances in the five years prior to admission. The only information asked for prior to this time concerned the topic of occupation; this was to gain a reflection of the residents' former status and wealth.

Alongside this information, a list of the main events leading to admission was compiled from the exploratory findings together with a list employed by Willcocks et al (1982) in their study of residential homes.

Elderly people were also asked to specify significant others in the process of their admission and to identify alternative directions which they could have pursued in the process. In a study of this nature, one of the difficulties proved to be exploring hypothetical options, particularly if people were not aware of what was on offer: they could only speculate on the feasibility of alternative situations.

Sources of finance highlighted in the exploratory study were compiled in the schedule and placed towards the end of the interview. Subjective and attitudinal data was also placed towards the end of the structured questionnaire. This centred around the mood of the resident together with their level of happiness and satisfaction with life in the private residential home

An unstructured framework was used to pick up more sensitive material such as acceptance or resentment felt by elderly people towards their situation, and the difficulties they faced in the process of admission.

Local authority resident questionnaire

Local authority residents were interviewed using an identical schedule to that employed in the private sector. However, additional questions, previously open-ended in the private study, were precoded (for example, one variable included an extra precoded category of 'who decided on this particular home?'). The state of admission - 'crisis' or 'planned' - was also pre-coded.

(2) The relatives' questionnaire. A formal questionnaire was not selected because the nature of the material collected in the exploratory study did not lend itself to this type of design. A semi-structured interview was again conducted with a relative named as significant by the elderly person and open-ended questions were asked. Several questions duplicated topics on the resident schedule in order to complement and provide a reliability and viability check on the residents' information.

Relatives were asked to give their perspective on the elderly person's life prior to admission together with the events they saw as influential in the process. Their role in the admission process was explored as well as their attitude and personal thoughts on the process. Finally, factual information on age, sex and marital status was collected to form a profile of relatives.

(3) Professional checklist. The professional perspective, included in another schedule, looked at the professionals' assessment of the situation in light of the resources available. Again, the checklist was designed to replicate topics covered by the resident and relative schedules. It also included a wider range of questions, for example:

- relationship, intensity and length of involvement with the elderly person;
- service request and response;
- assessment details;
- events leading to private care;
- alternatives available (this indicated what scope there was for alternatives to be realistically pursued);
- the experience of the admission.

During the interviews with social workers in the study of the private sector, the majority, unexpectedly and openly expressed their professional and political attitudes toward the privatization of residential services (Chapter Eight explores this in depth). As a result, two general questions were included in the local authority study to systematically elicit social workers' attitudes and views toward the private sector:

- How do you decide whether someone goes into a private residential home or a local authority home?
- What is your attitude toward the private sector?

(4) Interview schedule for the home owner. A valuable range of hitherto unknown information on the background of the home owner and manager, admission policy and practice as well as information relating to the admission of selected residents was provided by an interview checklist designed for use with the home owner. This looked at how the home owner assessed potential residents and why they rejected particular people. A broader picture of the home was also gained and included information on the philosophy of the home, its operation and the extent to which residents were given independence and choice about their life style. This enabled the process to be looked at from the 'gate-keeper's' perspective.

In addition, the researcher assessed each private home according to its overall image and philosophy (Chapter Three). A similar but shortened form of the home owners' checklist was used in the interview with the officer-in-charge of each local authority home visited. From the four schedules an outline plan of the research was drafted.

Interviews with other operators - for example, Assistant Divisional Organisers (Operations) in the local authority system - were considered, the purposes of which were to explore the policy governing residential home admissions in each division and to glimpse the general criteria used in the allocation process. Decision making in this sector, however, was complex and it was decided not to investigate this part of the local authority process because it was not directly comparable with the system operating in the private sector (which was the main focus of the study). Potential private sector residents were not required to undergo a professional assessment or 'journey' through a bureaucratic allocation system. The potential admission involved a direct relationship between home owner and elderly person.

The interviews: negotiating access

(1) Access to private residential homes. Although carried out under the financial sponsorship of Suffolk County Council, this was an independent

study and therefore access to private homes was direct, rather than through the county's registration officer. Initial telephone contact with home owners was also initiated under the auspices of the University. In retrospect, this independent line reassured home owners in such a way that they openly discussed the relationship they had with County Council staff.

Time was allocated to negotiate with home owners in case of possible difficulties in access. Over 90 per cent of home owners, however, expressed great interest in the research and were happy to be interviewed.

Home owners, selected from the stratified list of homes, were initially contacted by telephone and given details of the purpose of the study and the methods of data collection. Their co-operation was forthcoming at this stage in allowing access to their home and the residents they accommodated. Complete confidentiality was assured at this point, queries were answered and appointments made to begin fieldwork. Home owners were also asked to prepare a list of residents currently at the home and their dates of admission.

The next contact with the home owner came at the time of the visit. An interview was carried out with each of them regarding policy and practice and was followed by a discussion of the process of admission of individual residents chosen from the list (that is, those elderly people who entered within a period of one year prior to the researcher's visit).

(2) Access to residents. Caution was taken to ensure that the elderly people themselves had the opportunity to participate or withdraw from the interview. This involved the researcher, rather than the home owner, approaching each person to ask if they wanted to take part. Residents who were confused were interviewed under the same procedure.

Where possible, residents were interviewed in the privacy of their own room, unless they specified a preference for the interview to take place in the lounge or elsewhere. Time was allowed, in preparing the groundwork for these interviews, for people to move from the lounge to their room and to settle down before an explanation of the interview began. Interviews with elderly people were limited to one hour maximum and on average they lasted fifty minutes.

Access to residents in the local authority sector was not easier, despite the fact that the research was publicised in a letter to local divisional organisers with the blessing of the Director of Social Services. The information did not filter through to officers-in-charge or divisional area organisers. Access to residents was a particular problem in one local authority home where the officer-in-charge insisted that time be taken to contact next of kin to gain their permission to interview residents.

(3) Relatives. During the interview, elderly people were asked to name a 'significant other' who assisted them in the process of admission. The majority mentioned relatives and some mentioned relatives and professionals, who were contacted only with the permission of the elderly person (or home owner if they were confused).

Relatives were contacted by telephone and asked for their co-operation. Usually, face-to-face interviews were conducted with relatives in the comfort of their own homes. On average, these lasted one hour twenty minutes. When a home visit was impossible to arrange through inconvenience to the relative or the distance and time faced in travelling to see them, a telephone interview took place. Such an interview with relatives was difficult because it was problematic to give and judge acceptances of confidentiality. It deterred some relatives from recounting sensitive experiences and, in one or two cases, from the interview altogether.

(4) Professional access. Access was again negotiated by telephone and the majority of interviews were conducted over the 'phone, either because of the need to maximise the use of the researcher's time or because it was found that face-to-face interviews in the professional's office were more likely to be interrupted.

Coding and recording

(1) Brief shorthand notes were taken during the interview and written up on completion of each set of interviews. The precoded schedule was, however, filled in after each individual was interviewed and this was done in a separate room or space negotiated for the researcher's use with the home owner. A visitors' room was utilised in the majority of homes.

(2) Material was transferred from the schedule to a SNAP computer package.

(3) Comments from the semi-structured sections of the interview were transferred from the notebook to index cards, colour coded with regard to the topics covered.

Following the exploratory phase, such qualitative material from the interviews was transferred directly into a file subdivided into the topic areas, for example, life prior to admission, background events, significant others and so on.

Analysis

Analysis and data interpretation followed the stages of data collection.

(1) Quantitative data. A statistical package of analysis was used (SNAP version 6) to present frequency distributions from the precoded residents' schedule covering 50 variables.

Cross tabulations between certain variables were produced. Other mechanical functions - for example, chi-square were applied by hand and checked using a microstat package. In a secondary analysis of data some variables were combined and others recoded to give further interpretation to the data.

(2) Qualitative data. Data from all interviews was collected in such a way as to apply a grounded theory perspective in the final analysis (Glaser and Strauss, 1967). This approach not only provided an organizing technique for coding qualitative and quantitative data but was advantageous in allowing a 'deep interaction' with the data. Core categories and central concepts were

extracted from the data by comparing interviews, sentence by sentence, picking out the central related themes that frequently appeared. Grounded theory involved a circular process with the analysis forming the development of other core categories and themes. Although sentence by sentence analysis was time-consuming, it provided an exciting and fresh analytical framework to the data.

Response rates

A detailed list of respondents was updated throughout the study. The reasons for refusal were also listed and analysed at the end of the investigation.

(1) Representativeness. As a percentage of the total number of residents in private homes in Suffolk, 48 per cent (596/1240) were found in the 39 private homes studied. As a percentage of the total number of residents in private homes in the four areas - this was 60 per cent (596/998). At the time of the study (December 1985) there were 596 residents living in 39 private homes: 223 people had entered these homes in the previous year. As a percentage of the total number of residents in the 39 homes it was 37 per cent. The turnover rate of residents was 37 per cent.

Although residents who were interviewed arrived within the previous year, the analysis of the length of stay for residents in 34 of the 39 homes for 1985/86 revealed that, on average, they remained for one year and eight months in residential care. This data, therefore, not only represents recently admitted residents but also residents who were at least half way through their residential careers.

(2) Response rate of residents. At the outset there were a potential 600 interviewees in the private sector study and 360 in the local authority study. The target sample of private sector residents (for feasibility purposes) was 200 (90 per cent of the total sample population admitted in one year). The exact number of residents interviewed was 160 (80 per cent of the target population). Material was gathered on the remaining 40 from the accounts of relatives and professionals.

The following table illustrates the reasons for the 20 per cent non-response rate.

TABLE 2.3
REASON FOR NON-RESPONSE OF RESIDENT

Reason	Number	
Died	15	(data received from relatives)
Home owner refused access	17	(resident usually frail or confused/ confidentiality problem)
Resident refused interview	6	(or interview aborted at an early stage)
Resident unable to be interviewed	2	(Residents still in hospital after two visits to the home)

	40	

(3) Relatives. One hundred and twenty relatives were named as 'significant others': the remaining 80 did not name a significant relative in their process of admission. Five residents named more than one relative and although information was gathered on all relatives, only one per person was followed up which set the target figure at 115. Eighty-eight relatives were interviewed: therefore the response rate was 77 per cent.

A brief investigation of the 27 relatives not interviewed suggested they fell into four categories as Table 2.4 shows.

TABLE 2.4
REASON FOR NON-RESPONSE OF RELATIVES

Reason	Number	
Relative refused	4	
Resident refused access to relative they named	8	(relative was ill, resident felt relative would be annoyed)
Home owner refused access	5	(resident recently died/family problems/ difficult relationship between home and the family)
Other	10	(no known address/lived abroad)

	27	

(4) Professional response. One hundred and two professionals were named, but 22 residents named the same person as the 'significant other'. This reduced the number to 80 professionals, 75 of whom were interviewed (5 had left the area and were unable to be contacted). The response rate was therefore 94 per cent.

TABLE 2.5
COMPOSITION OF PROFESSIONALS NAMED AS 'SIGNIFICANT OTHER'

	Number	
Social worker	42	(interviewed in relation to their involvement in 71 admissions to care)
General practitioner/ district nurse/health visitor/community psychiatric nurse etc.	31	
Home help	1	
Occupational therapist	3	
Other	3	

	80	

(5) Local authority study. Interviews were obtained with 98 people (82 per cent = 98/120): 22 people could not be interviewed because they had either died (8), refused the interview (3) or, in 10 cases, the officer-in-charge refused access and, in one other case, the resident was unable to be interviewed through illness. Data on these unsuccessful interviews was collected through other means: for example, by interviewing relatives. The relatives' response rate was 81 per cent (42/52). One relative refused and the other 9 could not be contacted. Ninety-seven per cent of professionals took part in the study. The non-respondents were social workers who had left the department.

Table 2.6 shows that the data collected was on target, but not all the material was collected by interviewing the particular person in question. Where there were difficulties apparent in contacting and interviewing elderly people and their relatives, a process of substitution was considered but ruled out because the costs outweighed the benefits.

TABLE 2.6
SUMMARY OF INTERVIEW RATES

	Resident	Relative	Professional	Home Owner	All
PRIVATE SECTOR					
Potential/ target no.	200	115(1)	80(2)	39	434
Number interviewed	160	88	75	39	362
Response rate (%)	80	77	94	100	84
Data obtained by other means	40	27	5	-	72
LOCAL AUTHORITY					
Potential/ target no.	120	52	120	19	311
Number interviewed	98	42	113	16	269
Response rate (%)	82	81	97	84	86
Data obtained by other means	22	10	7	3	42

Total number of interviews = 632

(1) 120 named, but only one person interviewed
(2) 102 named, but 22 people mentioned the same individual

Reliability and validity of measures used in the study

1. Physical dependency scale. Because the focus of the study was on the process of admission and the main data collection effort was devoted to collecting wide ranging data relevant to this, resource considerations made it difficult to justify an excessively rigorous attempt to measure physical dependency. However, Booth (1985) asks whether severity rather than dependency perse should be measured.

A range of measurement scales were available to assess physical dependency which either required clinical assessments or were time consuming. The Crichton Royal Behavioral Rating Scale (Wilkin & Jolly, 1979) was considered but not used due to the length of time it would take to complete, which would detract from the main focus.

A simple measure of physical dependency adapted from Booth (1985) was employed (see Chapter Four for detailed analysis). The dependency scale used made a number of assumptions about the relationship between different measures. Each measure was given relatively similar weightings: for instance, a resident described as having limited mobility was assessed as having the same level of dependency as someone with controllable incontinence.

This scale was easy to use and not time-consuming, and was therefore advantageous. On the whole it worked adequately, although in a few cases, such as that of Mrs Westcott below, its major weakness was highlighted the physical condition of a person did not automatically affect their functioning in terms of mobility, continence and self-care as specified in the dependency ratings and may be recoded inappropriately as a result. Mrs Westcott said her arthritis severely handicapped her because of the pain she experienced, yet she was not wheelchair-bound, incontinent or unable to wash and dress. Consequently, her difficulties were not recorded in the dependent/very dependent group but in the independent grouping.

In defence of this, it can be argued that boundaries are always arbitrary decisions in any method of assessing dependency and on the whole it worked well.

The dependency scale used was not replicated in other studies and therefore comparison with studies of this nature was not possible. Even where scales were similar (Booth, 1985) very few studies looked at residents within the first year of admission, but looked at a 'within care' sample, spanning different years of admission. Also these studies rarely had a steady stream of admissions with the same degree of dependency and so comparison of a particular year group of residents was difficult.

Comparisons can only, therefore, be made within this study, that is between the two sectors. The method used, however, was thought to be perfectly reliable in fulfilling its main aim - a comparison between the residents in the local authority and private sectors in Suffolk. Moreover, it proved economical and efficient in its application.

2. A measure of mental state. The reliability of the measure used to record mental state has already been demonstrated by Wade, Sawyer and Bell (1983). The method was thoroughly tested in the pilot study and appeared reliable and replicable in the main study (see Chapter Four for the scaling). Some caution was used in classifying residents as confused, however, as some new residents displayed signs of disorientation in relation to their new and strange environment, rather than the onset of senile dementia.

3. Social class. Categorising social class on former occupation is particularly difficult when respondents are elderly: they may have retired thirty years prior to the interview and memory recall of a spouse's occupation may be difficult; the length of widowhood and lack of relevant occupational ratings when the occupations themselves were held in a very different occupational and industrial structure increase the problem. There is also the fact that social class ratings themselves may be irrelevant when based on occupations given up many years before.

4. *Mood/happiness and satisfaction.* The difficulties of measuring such subjective material have been documented in other studies (Peace, Hall and Hamblin, 1979; Bland and Bland, 1983; Fennell, 1986; Willcocks, Peace and Kellaher, 1987). Satisfaction levels, reported by residents, not only reflect the present environment and living circumstances of the resident, but also as Willcocks et al note:

> an accumulation of events which encompass their life in the community as well as the process of admission to residential care. (Willcocks 1987, p.123)

If this is true then the level of satisfaction may reflect the process making it difficult to disentangle satisfaction before and after admission.

Mood A recorded the interviewer's assessment of the resident's mood based on the picture presented by the resident from tone of voice, appearance, facial characteristics, willingness in response to questions and the way in which they described their life situation.

Mood B, in order to check ratings for Mood A, directly asked the resident whether they were hopeful about the future. In the final analysis there was a correlation between those who said they were 'hopeful about the future' and those who were assessed as 'jolly'.

The measures of happiness and satisfaction given their limited reliability anyway, proved reliable and valid, particularly when checked against relative and professional comments.

Limitations and biases in the data: points for further consideration

(1) Access to the homes. Although at the exploratory stage the possibility of widespread access problems was discussed, in the main study only one home refused after two attempts at contact. This was replaced by another private home. The benefits of a careful, diplomatic and natural style of approach, stressing independence, were apparent in the success and ease with which access was given. One can, therefore, feel confident in the sampling reliability of the homes in the four divisions used.

(2) Access to residents: the right to refuse. Some home owners and heads-of-home saw their role as gatekeepers and refused direct access to residents; this not only applied to confused residents. Some judged whether residents would contribute anything meaningful to the study and limited access to those who could 'talk well'. This problem arose in two local authority homes and one private sector home. In cases such as these a detailed explanation of the sampling procedure with the home owner or head-of-home was vital to help her understand the nature of the sample selection and bias that resulted if she selected the residents according to ability or 'chat skills'. This was particularly vital where there were a number of confused residents in a home.

Elderly people in the residential settings studied were *not* viewed as a captive audience but were given the right to refuse or accept the interview. The ease of gaining consent to interview an older adult because the person is bored, lonely and has no obligations so often mentioned in training manuals was not found in this study. Old people had better things to do with their time than answer the questions of a total stranger and although many welcomed the interview, it was not because it provided a temporary relief from boredom and loneliness.

The opposite view, however, was sometimes reinforced, not only by the visual picture of people 'sitting around the walls' in a communal lounge, but often by the conduct of the 'matron' or home owner. The persuasion and influence of such people was great and residents in some cases felt they had to answer questions. In the exploratory study one home owner walked into the lounge and announced that everyone was to be interviewed. One individual, who said later that she wanted to refuse, felt under pressure to accept and the quality of the response suffered. Another lady who was not interviewed felt offended.

Caution was, therefore, taken to ensure that elderly people were not pressurized by others into participating in the interview. At the outset of the interview, the nature of the relationship was explained to the home owner and resident. It was stated that this interview was different from a social worker/client interview and not a friendship with further visits, but one visit to ask a few questions regarding their admission. A research rather than a social work role was maintained throughout the study. Questions from elderly people relating to residential life outside the boundaries of the research were kept in the background.

After a careful and simple explanation, time was given for residents to 'mull' over the purpose of the interview and ask questions. Because of the constraints of time and memory recall of some elderly people, the majority of interviews proceeded immediately after this explanatory stage. In a few cases the researcher made initial contact to explain the purpose of the research and returned the next week to follow up with an interview.

Overwhelmingly, the interview experience was pleasurable for both researcher and elderly people involved. The majority of elderly people gave the overall impression of being relaxed and willing to talk and reflect on their process of admission. Mrs Fox, on completion of the interview, expressed how much she had enjoyed the opportunity to look back at events with someone, although initially she had been sceptical about any kind of research. Mrs Wright was very enthusiastic about being interviewed and, although a little forgetful during the interview, was anxious to carefully recall the events leading up to her admission.

(3) Confidentiality. Complete confidentiality was guaranteed at the outset of each interview. The issue of confidentiality was not taken lightly but well thought out during the exploratory phase. One particular problem focused on the nature of the research relationship. There appeared a potential conflict in keeping an independent line for the benefit of the research yet being responsible to one of the stakeholders - Suffolk County Council, the registering authority, whose Social Service Committee had approved the research.

The implications of discovering malpractice were explored in the field in one example. In the bedroom of one home, three ladies were found watching television, while another, in need of medical care, was clearly distressed by the constant noise. At the same home, a sign was displayed in the front porch requesting visitors not to 'feed the residents'. Although such practice was against principles spelt out in *Home Life* (Avebury, 1984), it was decided that confidentiality would be upheld and the registration officer was not informed of the situation, particularly in light of the fact that the home was due for its annual inspection within the coming month.

The purpose and implications of the interview conversation were outlined to all elderly people. Reassurance to residents from home owners was necessary on only two occasions, in one instance when an elderly person was worried that the researcher was someone from the DHSS who had come to tell her she had to leave.

Confidentiality was also an issue raised in interviews with relatives and professionals. Relatives sometimes voiced objections to the disclosure of personal information on the resident and were particularly concerned when such information had come from a confused resident. One relative interpreted the research as 'an unwarrantable intrusion' and requested a legal guarantee of confidentiality. Reassurance was given but the relative refused personal access.

The majority of relatives, however, responded to the request for information and were only too pleased to express their views on the process of admission and the difficulties they faced in caring for an elderly parent or aunt.

Surprisingly, professionals infrequently questioned the ethics related to parting with confidential information on patients and clients. Few questioned the authority or authenticity of the researcher and most were happy to give personal information on their cases over the telephone. Few practising social workers received any prior notification of the research, although a letter was sent to all area managers.

(4) Privacy. The situational context of the interview raised questions of privacy as well as confidentiality. As in any interview situation, the ideal was to be in an environment where there was a degree of privacy and comfort, with a relaxed atmosphere. In many homes this was difficult with 'busy' people such as cleaners going about their work or where there were other residents in the lounge. It was important for the elderly person to feel in control of their environment also, and this often meant assisting them to their own room. Such a journey was sometimes difficult for frail people, particularly if the walk down the corridor was the biggest daily task they faced. Time was also allowed for the elderly person to settle down before starting the interview.

The use of individual rooms was checked with the home owner or head of home at the start and, if this was not possible, a private (visitors) room was often put at the disposal of the researcher.

(5) Interviewing elderly people. There is no single model to apply in interviewing elderly people, simply because 'elderly' people as a single homogeneous group do not exist. Interviewing skills needed for researching situations of elderly people are no different from skills needed in interviewing other adult groups in society. The researcher brought personal assumptions and values about being old into the research design and style of interview and it was important to be aware of these. The interpretation of

the interview by the respondent within their own frame of reference and from their own value base was also important, particularly if a follow-up visit was required.

(6) Timing of interviews. The timing of interviews was crucial for two main reasons. Firstly, the distance between homes meant considerable travelling time; and, secondly, the institutional regimes intruded into the time available for interviewing - 4pm was a time to be avoided as well as times leading up to and immediately after meals. (However, in some cases, an invitation to lunch provided the opportunity to chat informally with residents and observe the 'ethos' of the home.) Times of general elections also intruded into the planned timetable, with canvassers in a number of homes interviewing residents regarding their voting behaviour and collecting postal votes.

Residents occasionally had guests with them and in some cases it was necessary to arrange alternative times and days for the interview. Such a situation often provided the opportunity to meet the 'significant' relative in the process of admission.

The length of the interview was crucial. For some people it was an unusual experience and possibly the first time they had been asked to express their views on the process of admission and therefore needed time to 'get into' the interview. The fatigue of the interviewee could also affect bias, although only one resident withdrew exhausted in the first five minutes. Interviewer fatigue also should not be underestimated, particularly when interviewing people who are depressed or going through a bereavement.

(7) The ability of elderly people.

1. Confused residents

Some elderly people had a limited capacity to retain information and had a very short term memory, even forgetting the identity of the researcher. Extra time was taken interviewing confused people as a degree of 'ventilation' by residents was advantageous in building up a picture of their current situation. The length of time between an event such as admission and the interview appeared important in terms of recall but the importance of an event - for example, a bereavement - sometimes took on overwhelming significance in the interview. Mr Scott said:

> 'In view of my wife's death I just live from day to day. I am completely absorbed with the thoughts of my wife not being with me'. (Mr Scott, The Suffolk)

A feeling of loss and anxiety took over in one case and in this situation the interview was abandoned and returned to later following a cup of tea and a chat.

2. Problems in communication

Some elderly people in the study had difficulty with their speech or hearing and again time was taken to make sure they understood the nature of the exercise. All steps were taken to help them in their communication and a few were reminded about their hearing aids.

Irrelevant information was also given as some people opened up their whole life with an undirected expression of feeling. This required careful re-direction and handling of the interview, particularly if the elderly person (or in some cases relatives) became tearful. Caution was also taken in the interpretation and analysis of data. Some people presented an ideal picture rather than reality (confirmed by home owner, relative and professionals).

A useful reference detailing further problems and challenges is given by MacPherson, Hunter and McKeganey (1988).

Conclusion

A stratified random sample of 200 private home residents was taken over four selected areas of Suffolk. Following the first stage of investigation, 120 local authority residents were interviewed to give comparative data on the process of admission into residential care. A high response rate was recorded for residents, relatives and significant professionals who commented on their role in the process. The successful rates of interviewing would suggest that the problems commonly associated with interviewing elderly people: for example, low response rates and limitations in communication, should not routinely be associated with interviewing this group of people. It is equally important to look at the approach and the style of interviewing and to prepare carefully in the initial stages of access negotiation.

Although there were limitations in the methodology, the advantages of the methods and analyses employed outweighed the pitfalls to yield a representative profile of residents and their process of entry into private and local authority homes over a one year period. The following chapters take up these themes.

3 Profile of private residential homes and their owners

An attractive feature of the private sector is its variety of residential provision. The ability to offer a number of homes, different in form, location and size to traditional local authority provision is a marketable quality. Creating a homely and caring family atmosphere is promoted by the majority of home owners as a major feature: others stress a firm medical orientation in their caring function. The image that results, however, stems from the style of operation within the private home, a style determined in the majority of homes by one individual - the home owner who, in general, is involved on a daily basis, holding the balance of power in the compromise between running a business and providing care services for elderly people.

In general, media coverage of the image of private residential homes has been condemning. Television exposures of practice or tribunal hearings have followed the minority of instances of bad practice that have come to light through critical events, like the trade union report '*The realities of home life*' (NUPE, 1986).

One or two examples of such practice have been translated and applied to the whole sector. It is a rare piece that finds some warmth or happiness in private homes. Most of the writing is dominated by judgements of damnation, with the private home resident doomed to be imprisoned in her room and in the conforming mould set by the home owner.

This chapter attempts to examine the image of private sector homes from the data collected on thirty-nine private homes in Suffolk - a sample big enough to provide a valid cross-section of the private sector in one county.

Following an account of the physical entity in which care is given and a profile of the home owners, the relationship between home owners and their enterprises is considered in terms of their motivations and style of operation.

A theoretical discussion concludes the first section.

The profile of private residential homes

The physical structure: function and form

Striking differences were found between the thirty-nine homes in their design and style of architecture. Much of the external appearance reflected the style of the period in which they were built. Five homes were constructed prior to the last century, with the majority (twenty- eight) built in the Georgian and Victorian era. A further five homes exhibited the style of inter-war building, with classic double bays, set back from the road.

Those built in Victorian times fell into two broad groupings, either semi-detached/detached set in their own grounds, or submerged in a street of terraced houses or hotels.

Although the style of architecture varied, the external image was in tune with the surrounding houses. Form and function were therefore not apparent and such a disguise of function was often cited by relatives and residents as an attractive (and marketable) quality of this sector.

Three of the homes in the study, located in the country (for example, Millbank) portrayed this quality by their isolation, while ten emphasised their function by advertising on a billboard outside the home. One home (The Suffolk) even went so far as to advertise all that was on offer to a prospective resident - a private rest home with stairlift, hot and cold water, and W.C. in rooms.

The question of form and function was sharply brought into focus by the number of adaptations and extensions that were needed to existing buildings in order to adequately carry out the caring function and to meet the registration requirements. Although in a number of cases, the external appearance was modernised, few adapted their approach to incorporate ramps and stairlifts to cope with wheelchairs. This was mentioned as one of the biggest initial headaches facing home owners.

The former function and origin of homes is shown in Table 3.1. Five homes served two or more functions prior to being used as a private home. Ten (26 per cent) of the homes were former private houses, some of which had been renovated and adapted in some way or another to meet the needs of elderly people by incorporating stairlifts and handrails. A marketable feature for both home owners and to residents was property designed to convey an ordinary small domestic setting and a homely image. The package inside, however, may be very different.

Former hotels lost out on this 'ordinary home' image, their size being the main detraction. Most of these properties resembled hotels, not small family homes, and were often set in a road of similar buildings which had kept their function as hotels.

Only one home was purpose-built (St David's) and resembled a traditional local authority style - set in a street of terraced houses, it was striking and obvious. Few elderly people gave away its function as a private residential home by sitting outside in any number, despite the hot summer days during the interviewing for this study.

TABLE 3.1
ORIGIN AND FORMER FUNCTION OF THE 39 PRIVATE RESIDENTIAL HOMES

		No.	%
Private house		10	26
Hotel		11	28
Private residential home		4	10
Purpose built		1	2
Rectory		5	13
Other:	teaching centre, country mansion, maternity hospital, sanatorium, children's home, farm, barn	8	21
		39	100

Location of homes

Critical in the relationship between form and function is the location of the individual home. Four areas of Suffolk were chosen in the study because of their contrasting levels of public and private provision: these are shown in Diagram 2.3. In two areas (Coastal and Waveney) there were high levels of private provision in relation to local authority residential provision. These areas were more likely to have a concentration of elderly people in private homes in contrast to the two other areas which were Ipswich, a large-sized town, and the other, Mid-Suffolk, an inland rural area with a dispersed population, with pockets of elderly people concentrated in small market towns like Stowmarket.

In terms of location, private homes were divided into six broad categories as shown in Table 3.2.

TABLE 3.2
LOCATION OF HOMES STUDIED

	No.	%
Rural green	6	15
Urban green	1	3
Coastal green	1	3
Rural grey	5	13
Urban grey	11	28
Coastal grey	15	38
	---	-----
	39	100

(i) **Rural green:** a home set in the countryside, divorced from any local facilities and neighbourly contact, generally isolated.

(ii) **Urban green:** a home located in a town but within access to parkland or set in its own grounds (giving a feeling of self-containment). A rural setting, yet in easy access to 'urban facilities'.

(iii) **Coastal green:** a home in an isolated location set on the coast, or small town along the coast, for example Southwold.

(iv) **Urban grey:** a home located in a built-up area, surrounded by similar style homes, no garden and with a feeling of centrality.

(v) **Rural grey:** a home set in suburbia - on the outskirts of a town or in small market town set in countryside, for example Stowmarket.

(vi) **Coastal grey:** homes situated in large coastal towns, in built-up areas.

A secluded country rest home described the first group. All six were isolated from any urban centre and two were built as country mansions. The brochure of Millbank described it as:

> A large country house built about 150 years ago. Situated in wooded parkland, where the trees have been made subject to a Tree Preservation Order. The gardens and grounds surround the house. The home enjoys wonderful views across a beautiful valley to the south.

The nearest town, however, was seven miles away and residents had to rely on the home owner's generosity to transport them to the nearest shops. The isolation of such homes was often played down in their brochures, with the emphasis alternatively placed on the aesthetic setting, very often accompanied by an attractive picture to seduce the potential customer.

The majority of homes, however (79 per cent), were set in 'built-up' areas - either in coastal towns or in a 'major urban service centre'. A necessary distinction needs to be made at this point between those with easy access to a range of facilities, such as shops, hairdressers, etc, and those isolated in suburbia. Twelve of the thirty-nine (31 per cent) homes were in residential suburbs. Those homes situated on the way 'out of town' were often in middle-class areas where property was cheaper than in central locations but again where access to a range of facilities required transport. In some cases the home was surrounded by hotels which afforded little opportunity for neighbouring.

The best balance of attractive situation and access to a range of facilities was captured by those homes located in small or medium-sized rural towns. The five homes in this group were within walking distance of their central shopping area and had attractive surroundings with, for example, views over the estuary or the broad. Another example is provided by Homewood, built in the seventeenth century as a rectory and set in its own grounds. It was in a street adjacent to the main centre covering a large hinterland. With roses around the door, it gave the appearance of being a homely cottage with no indication of function within, apart from being the domain of a private household.

Tangible features such as homely appearance through size and design of home mattered to both residents and relatives. The external appearance was a critical feature in the decision-making of residents and their families and a frequent attraction commented upon was the homely impression conveyed, mainly through size and look:

> It had an ordinary homely appearance which I liked.
> (Mrs Long, St David's)

> It's small, it's what she's used to and what she wanted.
> (Miss Comet, The Rectory)

The concept of home was important to many, not only in appearance but in location to the local shops. For others, the hotel impression appealed, especially with a location on the sea front with attractive views influencing their choice:

> It's lovely, you can watch the sea out of the window.
> (Mrs Bates, Limestone)

Some residents did not follow a path into a local authority home because the large institutional appearance reminded them still of the old workhouse system:

> I couldn't go there - it was too big, particularly after living in my cottage. It would still be the workhouse to me.
> (Mr Cord, St David's)

Those larger and isolated private homes within the depths of the countryside also gave the impression of an institution - one home was starkly situated in the middle of a field and noted as the only building around for several miles. Its isolation was accompanied by a feeling of quietitude and solitude, a place to disengage from wider society. Another was hidden along a country lane difficult to negotiate, in a valley surrounded by trees giving a dark and sombre appearance.

Homes conveying a homely image tended to be smaller with much more individuality in their exterior appearance: for example, one was adorned with hanging flower baskets. For the majority, in between these extremes, the exterior image was in harmony with their surroundings - bland front elevations disguising the caring function within.

Profile of home owners

Private residential homes in Suffolk presented a picture of a cottage industry; small scale business enterprises, predominantly family run, jointly owned and managed by a husband and wife team. This picture is not unique to Suffolk (Johnson, 1983; Jolly, 1986). There was no evidence of 'multi-national' or large company involvement in the provision of residential care (June 1988). At the time of the research, only one home was owned by a locally based company owning several homes in East Anglia and, in this case, the functions of owner and manager were separate. Nationally, there was also little evidence of large companies entering the market to buy up chains of homes (Phillips, Vincent and Blacksell, 1988). In the five years since their data was collected, the picture has changed. The petit-bourgeois model of small family-run businesses with relatively little capital is not the only model in operation. Large companies such as Wimpey and Retirement Securities Limited advertising through free papers like *This Caring Business*, have moved into the accommodation and care market for elderly people. Although this relates mainly to sheltered housing (Williams, 1988) there is no reason to doubt that the market will expand into residential care as in the United States. It will be a matter of time, therefore, before such business expands in Suffolk. Table 3.3 shows the structure of the homes sampled in Suffolk in terms of their management and ownership.

TABLE 3.3
OWNERSHIP/MANAGEMENT OF PRIVATE RESIDENTIAL HOMES

	No.	%
Owned and managed jointly (husband and wife)	30	77
Owned and managed by single person	2	5
Owned and managed separately	7	18
	--	---
	39	100

[Owner:	couple	4
	company	1
	single	2
Manager:	couple	4
	single	3]

For the majority of homes it was a family business: ownership and management went hand-in-hand for a husband and wife team. There were two examples, however, where one person carried out both functions of owner and manager and in both cases these were widows, continuing in the business after the death of their husbands.

Roles within the home

The particular roles of the female and male in the partnership depended on the size of the home as well as the number and roles of staff employed in the home itself. Although staff were employed in the majority of homes, many home owners provided the labour involved in caring for the elderly person and preferred to 'keep their hand in' by chatting to residents, supervising medication as well as keeping up with paper work. Three homes employed other close members of the family, for example a daughter or son, to carry out specific functions of tending, catering and administration or general care of the elderly residents. Relative input was in most cases considerable.

The small scale of the business was reflected in the division of labour within the home. Twenty six (67 per cent) homes employed husband and wife in segregated roles, with the wife predominantly taking on the caring tasks, the husband the administrative role (Table 3.4). Joint tasks of caring, administration and tending were illustrated by two (5 per cent) homes. Six (15 per cent) home owners exercised a segregated role, with the husband employed elsewhere outside the business as a builder (three instances), architect, farmer or lecturer, which helped to supplement the income from the family business. Three couples where the partners wished to work together, stated that they charged higher fees to supplement their income rather than find extra means of finance through employment elsewhere.

TABLE 3.4
SEGREGATED ROLES OF HUSBAND AND WIFE IN PRIVATE RESIDENTIAL CARE MANAGEMENT

	No.	%
Female carer/male administrator and financier	26	67
Female carer/administrator/financier (husband employed elsewhere)	6	15
Male and female - general tasks	2	5
	-----	------
*see Table 3.3	34*	87

Background of the home owners

Table 3.5 indicates the previous occupations of the home owners. The majority of proprietors, particularly the women in the partnership, had experience in the 'caring' professions, predominantly nursing (72 per cent). Of those with nursing backgrounds, however, few had experience of other appropriate jobs and consequently the orientation was medical. Only two out of the thirty-nine proprietors had a wide range of experience including financial and personnel management, catering and direct experience with elderly people in residential care, all essential skills needed to make a successful private home.

TABLE 3.5
PREVIOUS OCCUPATIONAL BACKGROUND OF PRIVATE SECTOR HOME OWNERS

	Women		Men	
	No.	%	No.	%
Nursing	27	72	2	6
Other 'caring' profession (including social work, the ordained ministry)	5	13	8	26
Self-employed	1	2	14	45
Local government	2	5	3	10
Law and Order	-	-	1	3
Other (including unemployed)	3	8	3	10
	38	100	31	100

The majority of home owners considered a nursing background to be vital and sufficient experience to carry out the caring task. A main worry for one home owner was her lack of nursing experience.

A number of home owners or proprietors had experience of managing their own business (36 per cent), although this was on a very small scale and very few had a background in managing staff groups of more than two people. A greater variety of experience came from the husband's former job - which ranged from farming, the grocery trade to the hotel business. Self-employed builders continued in their employment and saw their work as an additional asset to running a home, both in terms of income supplement and also when the need arose for structural adaptations and extensions.

TABLE 3.6
AGE STRUCTURE OF HOME OWNERS

	No.	%
Under 40 years	4	10
40 - 49	21	54
50 - 59	11	28
Over 60 years	3	8
	39	100

Most home owners, as Table 3.6 shows, were young and middle aged providing a variety of experience and background in the partnership which ensured a unique style of operation in each residential home. However, some element of nursing care was evident in most backgrounds and, as a result, the distinction between nursing care and residential care became blurred.

Length of operation as a private residential home owner

Very few proprietors claimed many years of experience in the job (only 18 per cent had over ten years experience as proprietors). The majority (41 per cent) had been in operation from three to five years with 23 per cent having less than three years experience in the business. Owning and managing a home for many was a relatively new venture as Table 3.7 shows, although some had experience as care staff in other homes prior to setting up in their own business.

TABLE 3.7
LENGTH OF OPERATION

	No.	%
Less than 3 years	9	23
3 - 5	16	41
5 -10	7	18
Over 10 years	7	18
	39	100

Minimum period 7 months
Maximum period 21 months

Motivation in becoming a home owner

A variety of motives were expressed by the thirty-nine home owners as Table 3.8 shows. Very few had one overriding reason to become a care home operator.

A number of home owners mentioned that the personal satisfaction they derived from working with elderly people was the prime attraction to this kind of work. Another considerable pull factor was the opportunity that the business provided for couples to work together. This often reflected their stage of family life as those owners over forty-seven years of age entered the business at the time when their children had grown up and left home. They were represented by the following comment:

> I'd got married and had my babies and decided I'd do this when they were a little older. (Greenfields)

Many younger couples found satisfaction in working together:

> We wanted to start again from nothing and work together as a team. (The Conifers)

TABLE 3.8
MOTIVATIONS IN BECOMING A HOME OWNER

	No.	%
Personal satisfaction	18	46
Business reasons (i.e. profit & investment)	16	41
Dislike of former job	14	36
Altruistic reasons	9	23
Stage of family life	7	18
Influence of third party	5	13
Elderly relatives	5	13
Redundancy	1	2
Other	1	2

n = 39 (up to two reasons were coded)

A major pull factor was the prospective profit and long-term investment that resulted from the business. Many home owners played down this reason and commented that financial rewards were not initially overwhelming or the major factor in their decision to enter the private residential sector. However, the business motive figures in 41 per cent of the sample.

Proprietors who talked readily about their profit margin set the attractiveness of the business in the context of their former employment:

> It provides more profit than the hotel business and more secure money for 52 weeks of the year. (Rosehill)

Only two proprietors suggested that making a profit was their only or primary motivating factor: both had previously owned and worked in other profit making businesses (restaurant and grocery trades) and saw private residential accommodation providing alternative profits (The Suffolk; Rosehill).

Another recurring theme was the dissatisfaction with a former job. Fourteen proprietors (36 per cent) were pushed into the business by this factor (three were former nurses working either in a National Health Service setting or another private residential home). They moved either from the public to the private sector (4 owners) or within the private sector (10 owners) in order to impose their own style and individuality on the job. One distinguishing and unique feature of private residential care is the impact and image that one or two individuals can create or change which may take many committees and levels of bureaucracy to achieve in the public sector. The red tape of the public sector was frequently mentioned as a reason for leaving local authority homes or the National Health Service:

> I've always wanted to do this and felt I could do a better job than remaining in the NHS - I hated all the red tape at the hospital. (St David's)

> Although I was Officer-in-Charge of a local authority establishment, I didn't have much say in the running - on what I could spend or on who were suitable residents to be admitted. In order to gain some freedom I decided to open up privately. (Crabfield)

Another home owner, moving from the public sector, expressed freedom from union pressure as a motivating factor:

> I was fed up of the NHS and the unions - you just couldn't tell staff what to do any more. (The Grange)

The title of 'Matron', together with the power and status as a result of being in charge were important to this home owner.

Former NHS nurses working in other private homes were motivated by thoughts of giving a better service if they set up their own business. Many felt that, as staff members in the Health Service, they had little power to suggest changes.

Differences were found in motivations expressed by the men within the partnership. On the part of the husband, it was boredom with a former job that tipped the balance for many.

An altruistic motive in setting up their own home was mentioned by nine owners (23 per cent): these people felt they could 'give something of themselves to the job' and two proprietors drew attention to their particular Christian philosophy which brought them into this kind of work.

A range of other motives were expressed. For example, Mrs Jones, a former nurse in the local surgery, knew many of the local old people whom she helped at home. Occasionally, she looked after elderly relatives, managing them in their own homes with a great deal of support:

> In the end I felt that I could do more if they were all under my roof. (Fenlands)

For another manager, the business was seen as a stop-gap before going into a private social work consultancy (The Suffolk).

The influence of a third party in encouraging potential home owners to set up in business in Suffolk was not as great as suggested by earlier research in this field (Willcocks et al, 1987). One general practitioner, assessing the increasing local demand, encouraged a proprietor to set up in business, feeling there was a shortage of such homes in the area. Another home owner was impressed by her sister's business operation in another part of the country and decided to turn her skills to the same enterprise.

Proprietors therefore came from a variety of backgrounds and experience with different skills and motivations for setting up in business. The nature of private residential care, however, meant that proprietors had to balance the right amount of care with the right amount of profit, as well as making their enterprise attractive to potential customers. Each proprietor was unique in arranging this.

Style of operation in private residential homes

Much of the literature and media coverage of private residential homes can be described as scaremongering - painting a picture of poor material standards and general predominance of the profit motive over and above the achievement of a caring environment: both the NUPE Report (1986) and '*The Granny Business*' (ITV, October 1987) are good examples of this. *The Guardian* (8.10.87) summarized these reports - showing old ladies strapped in their chairs for hours and old men eking out the last, humiliating days of existence - as 'utterly bleak' and 'an essay in the failure of democracy'.

Such condemning and judgemental descriptions focus their attention on a few private homes unfortunate enough to hit the headlines in recent years, and fail to extend their investigation to the sector as a whole.

The present research looked at the 'image' of homes from several different angles:

- the philosophy and style of operation within the homes as described by the home owner;
- general conversation with home owners regarding their attitudes to care;

- observation during visits to homes of environmental design and routines and of interaction between staff, home owners and residents;
- assessment of brochures and scrutiny of contract documents;
- interviews with residents; - interviews with 'significant others' in the process of admission - relatives and professionals who form an impression of the home, often prior to the resident.

In other words, the image was captured through interviews, observation and general assessment by the researcher.

The majority of home owners saw themselves offering independence, privacy and a caring and homely atmosphere in their home. On the basis of the absence or presence of each of these four separate variables, homes are described. The significance of describing each home's style of operation is to convey a general image of the private residential sector and not to judge what is good or bad.

Independence - dependence

Dependency is a socially constructed status rather than a biological one, created by the rest of society and imposed on those in elder years (Walker 1986). Goffman (1961) and others show that institutionalization goes hand in hand with dependency. Such research has led to conditioning attitudes towards elderly people which helped to shape policy and public expectation of their role and behaviour (DHSS, 1981a and 1981b). This perception of old age as a dependent stage in life can be embodied within the home itself, where staff are conditioned and residents conform to their expected roles.

The attractiveness of the private residential home, in this context, is its non-institutional feel, brought about through its size. But as Booth (1985) comments: 'changing the wrapper doesn't alter the contents' (Booth, 1985 p.206). The private home can still play a part in determining dependency amongst its residents. The routine of residential homes made necessary by their small staff, committed to an ideology of 'care and attention' can leave home owners less than enthusiastic about encouraging self-help and self-management.

The thirty-nine homes studied are described in terms of dependency.

Enforced dependency. There were examples found in nine homes of what would be described as 'enforced dependency'. The overt philosophy was summed up by one home owner's comment that 'we do everything for residents'. Embodied in this statement was a notion of 'disengagement'. The home owner saw herself providing a *rest* home for elderly residents to disengage from wider society. Two statements highlighted this:

> We are their servants and will pick up a hanky they drop on the floor... There's no such thing as risk-taking, we won't allow them even to make tea. (The Grange)

Control often fitted with an easier management structure in some homes while in others independence was difficult to achieve because of small staff numbers: One home owner said:

I'd have to follow him around all the time if I let him into the garden. (The Yarmouth)

Emphasised dependency. Rules and regulations governed the freedom of the individual and emphasised dependency in some homes. In one (The Suffolk), visitors were only allowed at certain times and all meals were cooked by staff. Very few residents in any of the thirty-nine homes had front door keys to give them an element of independence.

Encouraged dependency. There were several examples where choice and independence were stressed by the proprietor in conversation, but were not practised. Although one home (Millbank) encouraged residents to make tea and coffee and generally do things for themselves, to go to the nearest shop residents had to rely on the generosity of the home owner and the use of her car. Her attitude was patronizing, believing it was better to use her car than engage a taxi: residents, however, felt uncomfortable each time they wanted to shop.

Another example to highlight this came from a statement by a home owner:

> Residents have as much independence as they want within a structure that makes it workable ... I think, by the time you get to that age, you don't want to be making decisions. (Hillside)

Encouraged independence. Just over half of the homes in the study, however encouraged independence, individuality and autonomy.

Positive independence. This group included homes which allowed residents a degree of risk-taking and rehabilitation into wider society. Even the most physically and mentally dependent could be socially independent. This independence can be represented by the following statement of one home owner:

> Our philosophy is one of independence - we encourage them to bring their own furniture. In fact they are so independent, one lady of 100 years fell from her zimmer and later died - it's the risk you have to take. (Fenlands)

Research suggests that in theory proprietors allowed residents the right to take risks but in practice were very cautious in encouraging residents to be independent.

Public exposure - privacy

A number of homes emphasised elements of private space such as single rooms, but in all homes the main activity was forced to take place in the communal lounge or dining room. In twelve homes (30 per cent), however, it appeared that privacy was difficult to obtain.

A star example of public exposure was illustrated when, as a researcher, I was taken into a four-bedded room, without knocking or any introduction, to find one lady in bed with bronchitis and two others watching television. Another example of lack of privacy was illustrated when the home owner insisted on accompanying an elderly person on a visit to her general practitioner.

At the other extreme, privacy was respected when the individual could choose to remain in her room for meals and other activities. In one home (Fenlands) a resident's dog was even provided with his own kennel!

Twenty homes (51 per cent) laid emphasis on such privacy. One cannot generalise about the extent of privacy given to residents in this sector; many offered privacy in the form of double and single rooms but during the day emphasis was placed on communal living in the lounge. The home owner commented:

> Everyone has their own room. We have a certain time (12.30pm) when everyone has to be down for lunch.

Caring

This section presents a subjective assessment of the package of care on offer. The elements looked at were closely linked to the themes often picked up by the media - abuse of residents, attitudes of staff, assessment of interaction, commitment of staff to residents and general material standards.

Overwhelmingly, home owners demonstrated their caring philosophy in practice.

The majority of home owners and their staff (85 per cent) cared and gave an overall impression of commitment to residents. An example of a caring and thoughtful home owner who operated a key worker system is given below:

> One lady wanted to travel back to the countryside regularly in a taxi. I knew a local man who could take her so we invited him to have tea with her to get to know her before transporting her. (Fenlands)

Only six homes (15 per cent) showed a lack of commitment. In one example (The Lawns) scoring low on caring, there was a constant smell of incontinence, the furnishings were tatty, staff instructed residents and lacked sensitivity or empathy. A resident's room in one home was lined with white tiles.

Institutional - homely atmosphere

A rigid regime summed up an institutional home. Eleven homes (28 per cent) represented an institution by displaying multi-occupant bedrooms, regimented furniture, rigidly set meal times and little stimulation with 'people sitting around the walls'. This was accompanied by a strong emphasis on security - for example, in one home the door was bolted after someone had arrived.

Twenty-eight homes (72 per cent), however, did not lay any emphasis on rules and regulations:

The residents are encouraged to think of the place as their own. (Fenlands)

By observation most homes scoring high on this measure were small in size with individual rooms: they were also very homely and welcoming with home owners committed to maintaining each individual's private life.

Medical ethos - non-medical ethos

Six owners (15 per cent) with nursing training placed importance on the medical ethos and nursing style of care: for example, keeping staff busy with the physical tasks of caring and bed-making were emphasised.

In terms of image, seventeen homes (43 per cent) displayed a medical ethos in their operation. At one extreme home owners used labels such as matron, nurse and patient, wore uniforms and emphasised the physical aspects of caring. In one home (Greenfields) progress charts relating to pulse and bowel movements were completed daily.

A clear example of this medical ethos in the style of operation was portrayed in a sign on the front door of Greenfields:

> Would all visitors hand to nurses, food, fruit and sweets etc, before giving to patients. Diets cannot be adhered to if this is not done - THE MATRON

Such emphasis on nursing care constituted a powerful 'professional' model of caring (Phillips et al, 1988) and was attractive not only to the home owner but also to the prospective relative or resident, as in the case of Mrs Maloney's relative:

> I knew they'd care for her. It was evident they had nursing experience.

At the other extreme, there was little emphasis on anything medical despite the home owner's nursing experience: when the need arose for medical assistance nurses were called to the home. Seven owners (18 per cent) adhered to a social model, preferring to invite medical personnel into the home when necessary. Again no one state described the whole of the private sector, the main feature being its heterogeneity.

The image in the majority of homes was favourable. This was an encouraging sign as getting the balance right between profit and care, dependence and independence, often involved compromises. Independence, privacy and care were marketable qualities which were very often difficult to maximise in practice. Recent research (Booth and Phillips, 1987) has shown that small scale group living does not necessarily promote residents' independence: and other research (Weaver, 1985b) demonstrated that resident independence is difficult to attain given the complex nature of running a small-scale business.

Although the attainment of profit and care are compatible (Weaver, 1985b), the use of single rooms, giving independence and privacy to all residents, is less economical and makes the balance between profitability and independence difficult to attain. On the other hand, giving elderly people privacy may also be seen to demonstrate a lack of caring: for instance, elderly people found with hypothermia may be an example of lack of concern and care on the part of society, yet many such victims are found in the privacy of their own homes. The risks and rights of elderly people in any setting are difficult to balance (Norman, 1980).

Although the pursuit of profit imposed restrictions on the relationship between the institution and its residents, the pursuit of profit was not the prime motivating factor in each case. All homes had to break even or make a profit to continue in existence. However, the profit motive goes only some way to explain the differences between homes in their style of operation. The variety of styles of operation were determined by several additional factors, among them the experience and background of the home owner, their religious persuasion as well as characteristics of the residents themselves, to name but a few.

Despite such a difficult balance, the private sector remained marketable and could be seen in a favourable light in moving towards achieving the maximum self-respect for its residents.

Discussion

The opening section of this chapter described the profile of the thirty nine homes in the survey in terms of their physical structure and location. The proprietors' view of their function was described and, finally, the relationship between the home owners and their enterprise was subjectively assessed by the researcher in terms of the 'self-respect' of residents made up of the components of dependency and privacy.

It was demonstrated that form and location were vital concepts to address if function was to be understood. These three factors were also important in terms of the image conveyed to residents, relatives and researchers.

This chapter also illustrated that the private residential care sector cannot be described as a homogeneous sector because of the variety of provision and styles of operation it offers. Such variety was created not only through the pursuit of profit, which the majority of home owners had to achieve to be viable, but also through a range of other factors such as the pursuit of care and independence which were marketable and attractive to elderly people and their relatives in their selection of a private home.

Differences in styles of operation were also a result of the broad range of experiences and backgrounds of home owners, the extent to which they imposed their own ideas on running a business and caring for elderly people, the type of clientele they accommodated as well as the roles they themselves individually played within the home. Because of such a unique variety of styles, many proprietors saw themselves providing a real alternative to public sector provision extending choice to a range of different people.

Private residential care can still be described by characteristics alluding to small businesses, especially in the service industries: private homes were relatively new and were closely controlled by their owners. The motivations of such owners emphasised the desire for independence and pursuit of some personal satisfaction as well as some level of profit. There were a number of non-economic factors therefore indicating the typical entrepreneur was not solely motivated by a desire for profit maximization.

Another main motivating factor to set up in business was the opportunity to put one's own ideas into practice often after experience in the public sector. Most home owners translated this into providing a homely, caring environment (in contrast to an institutional setting in which a number had worked) replicating the services of a caring family. One home owner saw herself as providing 'a homely hotel with care', that is, accommodation with a level of care.

In the assessment of homes in terms of independence, privacy, care and homeliness (aspects which family living ideally provide) it appeared that 'professionally' re-creating 'the caring family' within the setting of a small private residential home was sometimes difficult. At home, most elderly people exercised a degree of power and control over their lives; once into a home, either public or private, the power balance in the relationship between the resident and home owner was clearly in favour of the latter. The style of operation adopted by some home owners clearly illustrated this. Some home owners reflected their nursing background in their relationships with residents (patient-nurse relationship) and in their style of operation.

Changing the form was found not necessarily to re-create domesticity: for instance, a minority of private residential homes set in small domestic residences placed emphasis on communal living and an institutional atmosphere - linked with a medical style of operation.

Such an enterprise as private residential care involved inherent compromises. Although home owners aspired to retain residents' independence, in practice they were seen to encourage dependency. It was also difficult to respect residents' privacy within the confines of available 'economic' space and a moderate caring and homely atmosphere. It appeared, therefore, that potential residents or customers bought into a sector of care that provided them with a level of physical care and a decent caring and homely atmosphere that afforded some independence. Overall, despite the variety of provision, a favourable picture of the private sector emerged based on the researcher's assessment and the opinion of residents and their relatives. Although there were homes which left room for improvement, on the whole the majority of homes provided 'professional care' within a profitable business framework.

Current trends, however, illustrate the erosion of the small business enterprise. Larger companies are finding a niche in the market of residential and nursing home care. The latest figures may show residential care for older people is at a turning point in its historical development. The slow strangulation and closure of petit bourgeois family run businesses as a result of the minimal benefits up-rating (November 1990) has seen the big business companies take over. Care of elderly people in the market with care being dictated by market principles rather than professional values has been achieved by Thatcherism.

Not only is the nature of residential care changing but the backgrounds of those entering the care professions changes accordingly - home owners need managerial experience with 'entrepreneurial flair necessary to ensure success' (*The Guardian*). The small scale family centred business with the owner in day-to-day contact with residents could become a thing of the past. Few job advertisements stress the importances of social work values and experience or even a nursing qualification.

4 Profile of residents entering private residential care

In order to understand the process of admission into the various private residential homes outlined in Chapter Three, it is necessary to consider what kind of resident entered both private and public sectors. This chapter looks at the characteristics of 200 residents in 39 private homes (1985/86) and 120 residents in 16 local authority homes in Suffolk during 1986/87. The aim of Chapter Four is to build a profile of the kind of person who entered a private home. It describes characteristics of residents in terms of age, gender, marital status and social class as well as their physical condition and mental state within the first year of admission.

The findings reveal that neither private nor public sector accommodated a unique and exclusive group of people. Residents with similar characteristics and profiles, mostly made up of physically independent widowed females in their 80's, were found in the two sectors. The extent of overlap between the populations suggests that there are two systems in operation (one based on need, the other on ability to pay) which compete for similar sections of the population, and to a large extent contain populations which are interchangeable.

Maud Blackthorpe provided a classic example of a woman who entered private residential care. At 87 years of age, after experiencing a fall, she 'put her name down for a private home' and kept in touch with the home owner until she was ready to enter. Her husband, formerly a local GP, died several years before. Although able to do everything for herself, she felt in need of some extra care and attention because she 'wasn't getting any younger'. At Gracelands she occupied an upstairs room and used the stairs to give her daily exercise. Physically she was capable of looking after herself and enjoyed life so much that she hoped to reach her 100th birthday.

Age

The average age of people who entered the private sector was 82 years (83 years in local authority homes). Men, however, entered private care at a slightly earlier age (81 years) than women (82 years). Average age revealed very little of the variety found in the private sector, so the distribution of age around the mean was analysed. In line with similar studies (Willcocks et al, 1987) and for the purpose of analysis, an arbitrary divide was imposed, splitting age into two categories: elderly people below 75 years of age were described as 'young' elderly, while those aged 75 and over were placed in the 'old elderly' category.

The majority of people were 'old' elderly with 83 per cent aged over 75 years (Table 4.1, Diagram 4.1, Diagram 4.2). Broken down by sex, 87 per cent of men and 82 per cent of women were over 75 years of age.

TABLE 4.1
AGE DISTRIBUTION IN PRIVATE AND PUBLIC SECTORS OF CARE

	Private		**Local Authority**	
	No.	**%**	**No.**	**%**
60 years and under	1	1		-
61 - 64	4	2		-
65 - 69	10	5		3
70 - 74	18	9		6
75 - 79	36	18		14
80 - 84	48	24		34
85 - 90	60	30		21
90 years and over	23	11		22
	200	100	120	100

DIAGRAM 4.1
AGE AND SEX DISTRIBUTION IN PRIVATE AND PUBLIC SECTORS OF CARE

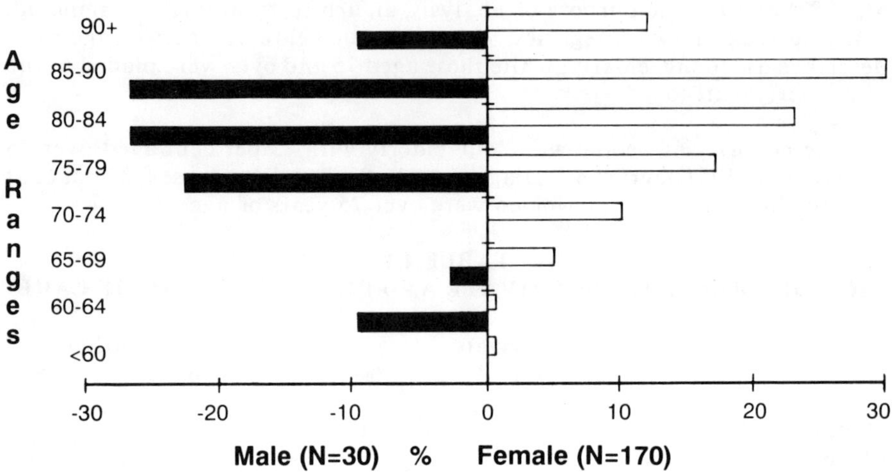

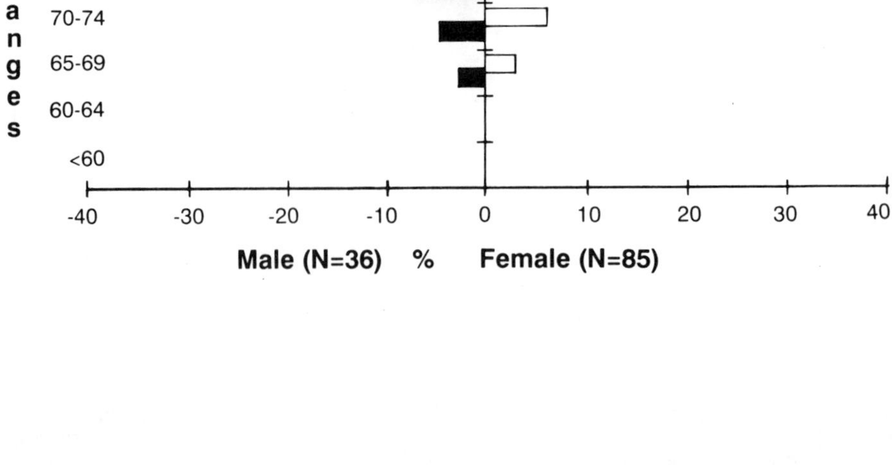

DIAGRAM 4.2
PRIVATE AND LOCAL AUTHORITY HOMES COMPARED
BY AGE AND SECTOR

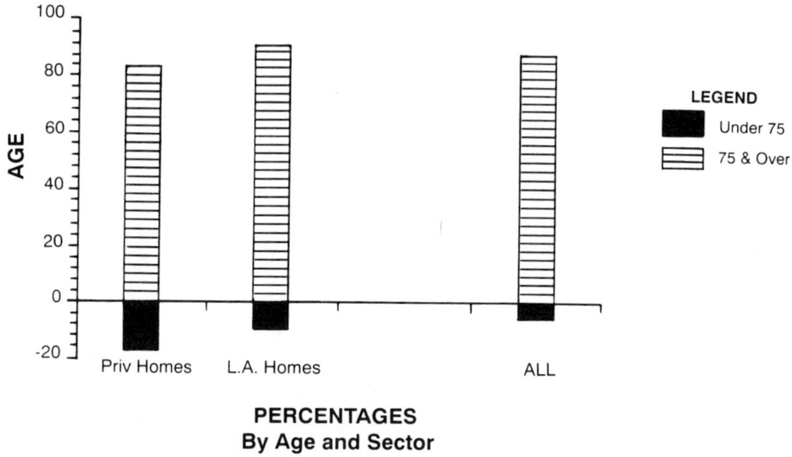

Gender

Residential care, in both private and public sectors was overwhelmingly female-dominated with 85 per cent of the sample in private care being women (Table 4.2, Diagram 4.3). Men were less likely to enter care than women, particularly those aged under 75. Among the 'young' elderly group in private care, the ratio of males to females was 1:7 and for the older group it was 1:5.

The imbalance was interesting as it suggested different processes at work for men and women entering residential care. It indicated that women, living alone, 'chose' to enter private care at a younger age, whereas men of a similar age were more likely to be cared for by their 'younger' wives at home, a factor which is well supported in the gerontological literature (Peace, 1986).

TABLE 4.2
GENDER OF RESIDENTS ENTERING PRIVATE AND LOCAL AUTHORITY RESIDENTIAL CARE

	Private		Local Authority	
	No.	%	No.	%
Female	170	85		72
Male	30	15		28
	200	100	120	100
ratio =	1 : 6		1 : 3	

Marital status

There were no differences in marital status between the private and local authority sectors. Table 4.3 shows that the majority of elderly people (74 per cent in the private sector) were widowed. Indeed, this highlights the traditional association between bereavement and need for care. Men in the private sector, however, were more likely to be married than women (Table 4.4). Only 3 of the men and 4 of the women, however, were still living with their partners in the same residential home; 8 wives and 6 husbands lived in the community.

TABLE 4.3
MARITAL STATUS OF RESIDENTS

	Private		Local Authority	
	No.	%	No.	%
Single	29	14		17
Married	21	11		8
Widowed	147	74		67
Divorced/separated	3	1		5
Not known	-	-		3
	200	100	120	100

The great number of widowed females who dominated this sector, can be explained by the longevity of women and the considerable loss of men after the second world war. Women have traditionally married men of similar age or older than themselves, which, given uneven life expectancy, makes it more likely they will experience widowhood.

TABLE 4.4
GENDER AND MARITAL STATUS OF RESIDENTS IN PRIVATE AND LOCAL AUTHORITY CARE

	Private				Local Authority			
	Female		Male		Female		Male	
	No.	%	No.	%	No.	%	No.	%
Single	28	16	1	3	-	17	-	19
Married	10	6	11	37	-	6	-	14
Widowed	129	76	18	60	-	72	-	61
Divorced/sep	3	2	-	-	-	5	-	6
Not known	-	-	-	-	2	-	-	-
	170	100	30	100	84	100	36	100

Social class

The social class of a resident was based on former occupation, which was classified according to the Office of Population and Census Surveys (Table 4.5). Occupation was defined as:

> the kind of work which a person performs, due regard being paid to the conditions under which it is performed. This alone determined the particular group in an occupation classification to which the person is assigned. (OPCS, 1980)

Differences in education and levels of remuneration were not shown.

The coding framework was taken from the classification of occupations. All residents were asked about their occupation together with the occupation of their spouse, and the information was checked with relatives. The man's previous occupation prior to retirement or the woman's occupation if it was dominant in terms of social class was taken as a basis for the categorization. If a woman was widowed more than ten years prior to the study, or single, she was categorized according to her own previous occupation. On this basis, a high proportion of women were grouped as 'housewives'. This created some difficulty in giving an accurate picture and as a result interpretation of the ratings should be treated with caution.

Despite this and other disadvantages (highlighted in Chapter Two) residents were assigned to the following social class categories:

I Professional	eg. lawyer
II Managerial	eg. self-employed, farm manager
III Skilled occupation:	
- manual	eg. missionary
- non-manual	eg. fire service supervisor
IV Partly skilled (other)	eg. hedger and ditcher
V Unskilled/unemployed/ housewife	

TABLE 4.5
SOCIAL CLASS OF RESIDENTS

	Private No.	Private %	Local Authority %
I Professional	41	21	8
II Managerial	26	13	2
IIIA Manual	45	23	38
IIIB Non-manual	25	12	35
IV Other	6	3	5
V Unskilled/housewife	35	17	3
Unknown	22	11	9
	200	100	100

The sample of residents in private homes contained predominantly 'middle class' people (Table 4.5) with 34 per cent previously holding professional or managerial positions. (Such occupations were primarily held by men). 'Working class' residents (23 per cent in the manual category) traditionally located in local authority homes (Townsend, 1962), were also found in the private sector having entered through the availability of supplementary benefit (50 per cent) or their own financial resources (33 per cent).

Financial circumstances (table 4.6)

Residents in the private sector were asked about their main source of funding: their ability to pay being a critical factor in their entry to this sector.

TABLE 4.6
PRIMARY SOURCE OF FUNDING IN THE PRIVATE SECTOR

	No.	%
Interest from stocks/shares and investments (not diminishing)	48	24
Diminishing capital resources	62	31
Relatives	8	4
DHSS (supplementary benefit)	68	34
Other, including insurance	14	7
	200	100

Over half the sample (55 per cent) were self-funding, either through interest from stocks, shares and investment or through diminishing capital stock, for example, sale of their housing property. In line with national figures (Bradshaw and Gibbs, 1988), 34 per cent of residents entered care through the availability of supplementary benefit. In line with the findings of Bloomfield (1986), therefore, it was not only extremely wealthy people or those from privileged backgrounds who were able to take advantage of private residential care.

Caution must again be taken in interpreting these figures because some residents were unaware of their source of funding. This was particularly true in relation to the source of 'top up' that several residents received. The low figure (4 per cent) attached to relatives' contribution may, therefore, be an underestimation of the number of elderly people supported by relatives. Other studies (Gibbs and Bradshaw, 1988) put the 'topping up' contribution of relatives at 34 per cent. This may be due to the fact that since 1986 the fees in private homes have increased (see Chapter Seven) and consequently more residents are having to rely on relatives for an extra source of funding. The ability to pay for private residential care was closely associated not only with the residents' social class, but also with their ownership of property.

Property ownership

The likelihood of people applying for private residential care was also governed in part by their ownership of housing. Townsend (1962) found that tenure and ownership of property were important in terms of whether people entered care.

TABLE 4.7
RESIDENTS' OWNERSHIP OF HOUSING

	Private		Local Authority
	No.	%	%
Self	98	49	28
Relatives/others	60	30	21
Local authority	23	11	29
Private rented	12	6	20
Housing association	7	4	2
	200	100	100

Half of those who entered the private sector owned their own houses at the time of admission and, therefore, had potential to enter the private market through the sale of their homes as Table 4.7 displays. Table 4.8 shows that people who were self-funding were more likely to have lived in their own property, with those on state support coming from rented accommodation.

TABLE 4.8
FINANCIAL SOURCE AND OWNERSHIP OF PROPERTY OF RESIDENTS IN THE PRIVATE SECTOR

	Owner-occupied		LA/private rented		Other		All	
	No.	%	No.	%	No.	%	No.	%
Self-funding	75	76	7	20	28	42	110	55
DHSS	17	17	26	74	25	37	68	34
Other	6	6	2	6	14	21	22	11
	98	49	35	17	67	34	200	100

Seventy-six per cent of those previously living in their own property financed themselves in residential care, while only 20 per cent of those in council or privately rented property were able to self-fund their placement. Many of these tenants (74 per cent) relied on DHSS support which provided them with the opportunity to enter residential care. Lack of tenure or ownership made a decision to apply for residential care more difficult to reverse and this particularly placed local authority sector residents in a vulnerable position.

The relationship between property ownership and entry to residential care was looked at in the light of social class. Wealth through ownership provided people based in different social classes with the opportunity to enter private residential care. Table 4.9 shows that residents from professional classes in both sectors were likely to own their own property. Those people in the manual classes in private care were also more likely to have owned property than those in the same class entering local authority care.

TABLE 4.9
SOCIAL CLASS AND PROPERTY OWNERSHIP OF RESIDENTS

	Professional/managerial				Manual/non-manual			
	Owner-occupied		Rented		Owner-occupied		Rented	
	No.	%	No.	%	No.	%	No.	%
Private	40	81	4	9	29	71	12	29
Local Authority	6	86	1	14	21	43	28	57
Total	46	90	5	10	50	55	40	44

As far as local authority residential care was concerned, greater percentages of people entered care due to homelessness and appalling housing conditions, without modern conveniences or running water.

Physical condition

The decline in physical health and ability to manage at home due to periods of illness has been well documented as one of the reasons for admission into residential care (Wade et al, 1983; Willcocks et al, 1987). Also well researched are the levels of dependency among residents in different sectors of care (Booth, 1985; Willcocks et al, 1987). Booth's classification based on a person's physical functioning and their ability to care for themselves was used in this study to assess physical condition.

Residents were classified individually on four simple measures making the dependency scale described in Diagram 4.3a. Scores were given to residents according to how they rated on each measure: for example, a fully ambulant person would score 1 on measure 1; if they needed help with bathing they would score 2 on measure 3, and so on.

DIAGRAM 4.3a
DEPENDENCY SCALE: PHYSICAL CONDITION

1. **Ambulant/disabled**

Not disabled/ambulant	(1)
Disabled/limited mobility	(2)
Very disabled/wheelchair bound	(3)

2. **Continence**

Continent	(1)
Incontinent but controllable	(2)
Uncontrollable incontinence/doubly incontinent	(3)

3. **Ability to wash and dress**

Complete ability without help	(1)
Needing help with bathing	(2)
Needing considerable help with daily washing	(3)

4. **Feeding**

No help	(1)
Sometimes in need of help	(2)
Always in need of help	(3)

Adapted from Booth's (1985) 'self care' scale

DIAGRAM 4.3b
AMALGAMATED DEPENDENCY SCORES

	Score	Range of possible sets				
Independent	4 - 6	MMLL	HLLL	LLLL	MLLL	
		2211	3111	1111	2211	
Dependent	7 - 9	HMMM	HHLL	HMHL	MMMM	HMML
		3222	3311	3231	2222	3211
Very dependent	10 -12	HHHH	HHHM	HHHL	HHMM	HHML
		3333	3332	3331	3322	3321

These scores were amalgamated (diagram 4.3b) to give an overall measure of dependency. Residents were described as 'very dependent', 'dependent' or 'independent' according to their level of mobility, continence and their performance at washing, dressing and feeding.

Group 1 consisted of people whose combined scores of 4 to 6 classified them as independent on at least three of the measures and described them as ambulant (with or without aids, but without personal assistance), continent and fully capable of dressing, feeding and washing themselves.

Those who were dependent (7 to 9 scores) had at least 2 of the following - limited mobility, controllable incontinence, were in need of help with bathing and sometimes help with feeding (none of the Suffolk sample needed help with feeding in this second category). Residents who scored 10 to 12 points came into the very dependent category: that is, they were classified as very dependent on at least 2 of the 4 measures. The limitations of using such measures were discussed in Chapter Two.

TABLE 4.10
PHYSICAL CONDITION: DEPENDENCY OF RESIDENTS IN RESIDENTIAL CARE

	Private No.	Private %	Local Authority %	All %
Very dependent	28	14	22	17
Dependent	54	27	26	26
Independent	16	58	50	55
Not known	2	1	2	2
	200	100	100	100

The dependency scale was used across both sectors. Table 4.10 illustrates that residents in both sectors were independent. Around half the people who entered residential care (58 per cent in private) were not physically dependent. This was similar to the distribution of dependency found by Booth (1985) where the largest percentage of residents were described as independent on all four dependency scales used.

Variations within the private sector can be seen when gender and age are considered. Men were more dependent than women (Table 4.11), particularly those men concentrated in the younger age group. The group of men who entered private homes in need of physical care were mainly those who were married (63 per cent of the 11 married men were classified as dependent or very dependent). This suggests that one reason for men entering care was the inability of their wives to support them at home. Mr Robinson, described below, provides an example of this.

TABLE 4.11
PHYSICAL CONDITION AND GENDER OF RESIDENTS ENTERING PRIVATE RESIDENTIAL CARE

	Female		Male	
	No.	%	No.	%
Very dependent	22	13	4	13
Dependent	39	23	14	47
Independent	102	60	12	40
Not known	7	4	-	-
	170	100	30	100

Behind these figures and descriptions of dependency were residents who should not be lost from the study. Three illustrations, one from each dependency category, are included below.

Miss Strict (aged 103, independent widow in private care)
Miss Strict had recently moved to Fenlands after a lifetime residing in the same house. She described herself as a 'simple lady living an ordinary plain life'. Although she never had a family and lived alone for many years, she was seldom lonely and was kept very active with church activities. Apart from slight deafness, Miss Strict was 'very much with it'. She had an excellent memory and held very strong views on different aspects of life. Her admission to Fenlands was precipitated by a fall at home, when she broke her hip and had to be admitted into hospital. In discussing her future with the hospital social worker she refused home help and other formal supports. Although she had good neighbours, she did not want them to feel responsible for her and decided that it was time she 'made a move into a home'. Fenlands was situated at the bottom of the street where she lived and, along with the locally born home owner, was well known to Miss Strict. She was well known herself - being the oldest resident in the town. At Fenlands, she settled quickly into her single room on the first floor, was very active both within and outside the home, and kept up her social contacts. (Dependency scale score = 4; ambulant/continent/complete ability to wash, dress and feed herself.)

Mr Robinson (aged 78, very dependent married man in private care)
Following a very active life engaged in running his own business, Mr Robinson suffered a stroke four years ago which left him wheelchair bound, incontinent and in need of considerable help with dressing and washing. He sometimes needed help with feeding. Although he employed several private nursing aides at home his wife felt she struggled to cope, Mr Robinson being

a large man and 'difficult to handle'. Mrs Robinson, at the end of her tether, approached Fenlands knowing that the home owner - who had previously nursed her husband - would be able to physically care for him.

Mr Robinson kept very much to his room. Although on the ground floor, there were steps to the dining room and so he used his large single room as a bed-sitter and diner. It had a pleasant outlook over the garden and duck pond and had a private entrance. His wife visited daily and other residents often joined him in his room for social gatherings and prayer meetings. (Dependency scale = 11; wheelchair bound, uncontrollable incontinence, needing considerable help with daily washing, sometimes help with feeding.)

Mr Nicholls (aged 74, dependent widower in a local authority home)
'Everyone says I've blossomed since I arrived, and I have. My life was restricted before and I needed a lot more attention when I was at home. Now with the space I can use my electric wheelchair and I can do a lot more for myself. I now only sometimes need help with dressing and its usually just my socks. It wasn't my decision to come, I had no option, but I'm better off here'.

Mr Nichols lived in sheltered accommodation for 5 years following his wife's death. His physical condition deteriorated to the extent that he slept fully clothed in a chair. He received help with cooking as his arthritis severely disabled him from lifting. He felt the warden put pressure on him to leave as his 'water trouble had become so bad'. The final straw came when the home help fell ill: 'the warden didn't want to know me', he said. (Dependency scale = 8; wheelchair bound, incontinent but controlled, needing help with bathing, no help with feeding.)

The concept of independence, describing the majority of people who entered private care, is highlighted by comparing residents in the local authority sector. Here too, as Table 4.10 shows, residents were independent. The overuse of the concept of dependency in residential care can also be seen when the physical condition and mental state of each individual was combined to give an overall score of dependency. Table 4.12 presents a comprehensive picture, covering those who were very physically dependent and always confused to those who were independent and never confused.

TABLE 4.12
SUMMARY CLASSIFICATION OF DEPENDENCY

	Private No.	Private %	Local Authority %
Group 1: severely dependent			
HH Very dependent/always confused	2	1	10
HM Very dependent/sometimes confused	8	4	5
MH Dependent/always confused	2	1	12
	12	6	27
Group 2: moderately dependent			
MM Dependent/sometimes confused	16	8	5
LH Independent/always confused	30	15	16
HL Very dependent/never confused	14	7	7
	60	30	28
Group 3: independent			
ML Dependent/never confused	32	16	10
LM Independent/sometimes confused	26	13	8
LL Independent/never confused	58	29	26
	116	58	44
[Not known	12	6]	
Total sample number =	200		

The similarity between the two sectors was striking. Although the local authority accommodated a greater section of the 'heavy end of the market' (Group 1, Table 4.12), the two sectors were alike in caring for predominantly independent residents and similar percentages of moderately dependent people (30 per cent private, 28 per cent local authority).

This indicates that there was considerable overlap in the kind of resident that each sector selected; for example, someone who was physically independent, but always confused and to a lesser extent someone very physically dependent but never confused, like Mr Robinson. 'Dependency' is certainly an over-rated concept in terms of planning for the typical needs of elderly people in both sectors. There has often been public concern that the private sector 'hives off' residents who are totally independent, leaving those confused, incontinent and in 'real' need of high levels of care and supervision to the struggling public sector, swamped by existing high levels of dependency (see Literature Review). The evidence from this research, however, points to the fact that it is not only the private sector which caters for the independent resident but also the local authority sector, which has several implications for the routes into residential care.

Mental state

The state and level of confusion was also looked at in detail. The interviewer's assessment of mental state was based on observation of the resident, communication skills and orientation, followed by a statement from the home owner on the residents diagnosis and stage of senile dementia, if any. The limitations of using such a method were discussed in the Chapter Two. Confusion was rated on three levels.

1. 'Always confused'

included residents who were totally disorientated in time and place; were unable to communicate during the interview and - based on the home owner's evidence - at most other times and residents with no short or long term memory recall. This group included people who suffered from a state of advanced senile dementia.

A person in Group 1 was Mrs Aaler who was admitted to a local authority home. For a number of years there had been several anxious reports of Mrs Aaler wandering and leaving the gas on in her flat. As a result of a gas explosion she was admitted to the local psychiatric hospital under a guardianship order where she was diagnosed as suffering from advanced senile dementia. Her complete lack of conception regarding time or place was symptomatic of her advanced dementia and, when admitted to the home, she was described as a problem because of her continual wandering, constant wailing and physical abuse of other residents.

2. 'Sometimes confused'

included residents who were sometimes disorientated in time and place or had some difficulty with memory recall.

During the interview, Mrs Crisp (Group 2) experienced difficulty in recalling her journey into residential care. Her sister, stated that she had been found on the floor confused and hallucinating. She was not feeding herself or getting regular sleep. Mrs Crisp was aware of her environment, although she had periodic problems in recalling specific day to day details.

3. 'Never confused'

comprised of a number of residents who were mentally alert with good memory recall and were totally aware of their environment and situation.

With advancing age, Mrs Fox (Group 3) felt it was time to look for a home and so engaged her solicitors to investigate the field of residential care and plan her admission. At The Beeches she was able to continue life as before with the additional care she needed. All day to day and financial matters were decided by Mrs Fox who enjoyed life to the full.

From Table 4.13 it is clear that the largest group in private residential care were mentally alert and never confused. Over half (53 per cent) of the sample were never confused, followed by a quarter (26 per cent) who were sometimes confused and a fifth who were always confused.

TABLE 4.13
RATINGS OF CONFUSION: RESIDENTS IN PRIVATE AND LOCAL AUTHORITY RESIDENTIAL CARE

	Private		Local Authority
	No.	%	%
Never confused	106	53	43 [41]
Sometimes confused	52	26	18 [18]
Always confused	38	19	37 [32]
Not known	4	2	2
	200	100	100

[ ] = percentages *excluding* local authority EMI home.

There were no significant statistical differences in gender or age. Half the men and women, and half the 'old' and 'young' categories of elderly people were never confused. Differences were evident, however, in the marital status of women (Table 4.14): 60 per cent of married women in private care were confused. This again suggests that the inability of a carer - particularly a husband - to support an elderly person at home, led to the need for residential care.

TABLE 4.14
MARITAL STATUS OF WOMEN AND THEIR LEVEL OF CONFUSION IN THE PRIVATE SECTOR

	Single/Divorced		Married		Widowed		All	
	No.	%	No.	%	No.	%	No.	%
Never confused	21	68	3	30	65	50	89	52
Sometimes confused	7	22	1	10	34	26	42	25
Always confused	3	10	6	60	25	19	34	20
Not known	-	-	-	-	5	4	5	3
	31	100	10	100	129	100	170	100

Mrs Waverley illustrated the type of person in this group. This lady (aged 86) was cared for by her husband who was struggling to keep her at home. She suffered senile dementia for a considerable number of years, was deteriorating physically and becoming incontinent. Although short stays at a local home provided her husband with some relief, they exaggerated her confusion. She was eventually admitted to hospital and then to a private home.

Although the majority of residents were lucid, this illustrates that confused people were not totally excluded from this sector. Confused people were found in three specialist homes for the 'elderly mentally infirm' which fell within the random sample. The total sample populations of these three homes suffered from some form of mental disorder, particularly advanced levels of confusion and psychotic breakdown, often accompanied by outbursts of 'bizarre' behaviour (see Chapter Five).

In eight of the 39 private sector homes (20 per cent) there were no confused residents. This partly reflects the home owners' perception of their role and function (illustrated in Chapter Seven) in caring for physically frail, rather than confused elderly people, which again was reflected in the fact that in 62 per cent of private homes over half the sample were mentally alert.

Differences between residents in private and public residential care

1. Level of confusion

Confused people, particularly those with advanced forms of dementia, were more likely to enter local authority homes: 55 per cent of the residents suffered from confusion as Table 4.13 illustrates. Not only were there significantly higher percentages of confused people in the public sector but there was a greater spread of confused residents between homes. All homes in the local authority sector contained residents suffering from some form of confusion. In thirteen (81 per cent) of these homes, half or more of the residents interviewed were confused. Even excluding the one specialist EMI home in the sample does not distort the main finding i.e. that a greater number of confused residents were found across the whole sector (Table 4.13, column 3).

The difference between the sectors is interesting because it indicates that those admitted to private care entered a different environment to those who entered local authority residential homes, where they were more likely to mix with people suffering a variety of mental disorders, particularly senile dementia. In reality it was not only the levels of confusion that were important but the behavioral and management difficulties that accompanied this deterioration in mental state. In the description of confused residents, the local authority sector was littered with accounts of residents displaying chaotic living patterns prior to admission, behavioral problems and 'bizarre' behaviour while in care. Below, a random selection of two case studies from the public sector illustrates the evidence of confusion linked with difficult personality in this sector.

Mr Page was admitted because he was considered a fire hazard, having several times set fire to himself and his house. Following admission to a local authority home he constantly displayed aggressive behaviour and was paranoid about the staff. His behaviour was sometimes escalated by frequent grand-mal fits.

When in residential care, **Mrs Jones** often lay on the lounge floor or took to her bed shaking and sometimes refused to eat. She possessed bizarre ideas of death and was described by the home owner as having a very 'inadequate personality'. After several assessments it was decided that she was in need of specialist handling in an elderly mentally infirm unit.

Similar profiles of residents in advanced states of confusion or suffering psychotic breakdown were only found in the three specialist homes in the private sector (case studies below). Apart from these homes, other private homes cared for residents with conditions such as nervous breakdowns (4), depressive illnesses (3) and sufferers of amnesia (6).

Home 1 - The Suffolk. Mrs Smith displayed eccentric and difficult behaviour. Her dementia released her sexual inhibitions and her behaviour was described as intolerable. Mrs West was left confused and incontinent following a stroke. Her behaviour was aggressive and abusive and as a result the home constantly kept the doors locked to stop her wandering.

Home 2 - Crabfield Hall. Mrs Talbot was hyperchondriacal and gradually 'went to pieces', making panic phone-calls and bizarre suggestions.

Home 3 - Willow House. Mrs Wade had always been a little eccentric, but her confusion exaggerated this and she very easily became 'uncooperative'.

2. Social class

Significant differences between the two sectors also existed in terms of social class (Table 4.5). In comparison with the private residential sector, in which there were more people from social class I and II, the local authority sector was heavily represented by residents from social classes IIIA and IIIB. Seventy-three per cent were from manual and non-manual occupations, compared to 35 per cent of residents who entered private care.

It is also important to note two further points: there were reduced numbers of housewives in the local authority sector (only 1 per cent of housewives in the public sector compared with 14 per cent in the private sector) which is explained by the fact that there were more women previously employed in this sector.

The 'working class' residents (23 per cent) found in private care were more often akin to the middle class resident in private care and were different in profile to the sample of residents who entered public sector care. We are, therefore, talking about one population in private care and not two separate groups - one middle class and another working class with profiles resembling those in local authority homes.

The difference in social class clearly divides the two populations and demonstrates that the ability to pay partly based on wealth through (own or spouse's) previous occupation is a major factor in gaining entry to the private sector. Related to this, the differences in ownership were also significant as highlighted in Table 4.7. This confirms the argument of Bessell (1983b) that the growth in private residential care is due to long-term trends towards increased home ownership and occupational pensions.

In summary, the two sectors were alike in major respects - they catered for similar people. The significant differences between the two populations were found in relation to the level of confusion, ownership and social class of residents. Other differences were marginal.

Discussion: What kind of people entered private residential care?

Although 'elderly people' - a group of people spanning the age range of 60 to 100 plus cannot be described as a single homogeneous group of people, the literature review (Chapter One) highlighted evidence to suggest that particular types of elderly people entered residential care (Tobin & Lieberman, 1976).

This chapter showed that there were a number of similarities in the profile of elderly people coming into residential care, irrespective of the care sector into which they were admitted.

'Typical' examples can be found among the women who entered residential care, widowed and in their early 80's. Such women were physically independent, not in need of regular assistance with washing, dressing and feeding; they were continent and were mobile. The new residents were generally mentally alert, with some memory recall and good communication skills. A majority of the women were formerly housewives, prior to the retirement of their husbands, who probably held local manual jobs typical of the region, or followed a career in certain professions. The majority of people, therefore, who entered private residential care can be described as 'typical older members of society'.

The interesting finding in this chapter is that a large part this description fits the residential care population of the two sectors. Both public and private residential care homes were dominated by widowed females in their 80's who were physically independent. The critical differences that were evident between sectors were in mental state (Table 4.13), social class (Table 4.5) and property ownership (Table 4.7).

The finding illustrated above is important because it means that there were very similar people entering two different systems, one based on need and the other on ability to pay. This suggests in theory that each sector could cater for the residents of the other, which also implies there existed a great deal of duplication between sectors. In other words, the private sector could replace the local authority sector in providing residential care for elderly people given increased funding.

A closer look at the significant differences between the sectors, ie in relation to confusion and social class reveals that the private sector did not totally exclude any particular group. Although the majority of people in the private sector were mentally alert, there was a significant minority of confused residents (Table 4.13). In terms of social class also, there existed a large percentage of 'working class' (social class III) residents who entered through available DHSS funding or their own personal means.

The private sector could, therefore, expand its provision for such groups, particularly if DHSS funding expanded alongside. The ability to pay was the crucial factor in the private sector and, unless funding is available, access for all groups to the private sector is limited.

There was also no evidence that young and healthy elderly people chose to go into private care or that the more severely dependent had no option but to enter the public sector (Table 4.12). This not only demonstrates that the private sector caters for similar levels of dependency but lends support to the argument for public sector replacement. Although this study did not look at 'need' for residential care, the similarities between sectors suggests that despite being based on different criteria (ie. a professional definition of need as opposed to ability pay), the processes operated equally sufficiently to select those people in similar need.

The marginal differences that were evident in profiles reflected the differences in these processes. For example, a professional definition of need for residential care may be reduced if support systems such as caring wives exist. This may go some way to explain why more married men were found in the private sector, where the abilities of the wife to cope were evaluated by the carer herself rather than a professional.

Because of such similarity, demographic features and profile characteristics alone do not offer sufficient explanation as to why some people went into private care and others into local authority residential care. The difference between the two sectors on social class and ownership which influenced ability to pay did go some way to explain why some people were able to enter the private sector. The reasons why people enter private residential care, how they enter and who selects them in the process are, therefore, discussed in subsequent chapters.

5 The journey into residential care

Chapter Four demonstrated that two sectors of care competed for similar sections of the population. The majority of residents in both private and public sectors were female, aged over 75, widowed, physically independent and mentally alert.

From the differences in profile, in relation to social class, ownership and mental state, there was evidence that a distinct group emerged in each sector. Elderly people, formerly in managerial and professional positions during their working life and thus more able to pay for care were more likely to be found in private homes. The ability to pay was a vital factor in entry to this sector. In contrast to the private sector, greater numbers of confused people were likely to reside in local authority homes. However, the overall similarity and the few differences in profile did not lead to a complete explanation of why some elderly people entered private and others entered public sector residential care.

Chapter Five attempts to answer this and looks at the journey into residential care by tracing the sequence of movements of elderly people from the background of the admission through to the final entry: it covers their reasons for admission, their routes into care and source and nature of entry. The chapter describes the kind of process as seen by residents, relatives and professionals and looks at whether similar types of people, in the five years prior to entry, went through a particular process to arrive at their destination and whether the different groups highlighted in Chapter Four entered via similar or different processes.

Describing the journey into residential care as a 'process' conjures up the image of a series of actions, flowing uninterrupted until the elderly person is admitted into a residential home. Chapter Five, however, shows that the process of admission was triggered very often by circumstance and not necessarily through a planned choice.

The sequence of care: conclusions

The private sector was made up of a large number of elderly people such as Mrs Giddens below who used the proceeds from the sale of her house to enable her to move into a private residential home. The majority, despite living alone and receiving little help or contact from any formal sources of support such as GPs and social workers, were well supported by various members of their family. Relatives coped with a variety of levels of physical and mental dependency to such an extent that when they were unable to continue in such a caring role, the only alternative for the elderly person was to seek admission into residential care. The influence of relatives to seek an alternative network of care was also a deciding factor leading to admission.

A similar process operated for those who entered local authority homes, although a greater percentage of residents entered care because of a deterioration in their mental state. This was particularly the case where families were unable to provide those suffering senile dementia with the necessary level of care to keep them at home, despite a number of them receiving local authority domiciliary services.

Life prior to admission

Living circumstances

During the five years prior to admission, the 82 per cent of residents lived in ordinary residential settings in the community (Table 5.1).

TABLE 5.1
TYPE OF RESIDENTS' FORMER HOUSING

	Private No.	Private %	Local Authority %
House	88	44	50
Flat	40	20	14
Bungalow	36	18	20
Other (caravan, institution)	36	18	16
	200	100	100

Apart from a number of the remaining 18 per cent who already lived in other residential homes or hospital, the majority of people faced a move from the community to an institutional setting, a change from living in a house or flat to one room, and from an environment which emphasised private space to a situation where communal space was the norm.

For many people leaving a familiar environment and adapting to a new setting brought with it the psychological feelings of loss, separation and abandonment. For example, Mrs Peters (The Limes) said:

> 'I just wasn't happy coming here at first - I felt my niece just abandoned me. I wish I'd not given up my home'.

Mrs Peters had difficulty managing due to restricted mobility and recognised the time had come when she could no longer continue at home.

Relatives reinforced this view. In hindsight, relatives, themselves, sometimes felt anxious and guilty about the move:

> She'd prefer a place of her own - she thinks because we got her in here that it's our fault. She doesn't make any effort to understand how we feel. (daughter of Mrs Price, The Windmill)

Another resident, Mrs Grosvenor, who was very bitter about her admission to Underwood, conveyed a feeling of hopelessness as a result of being completely ignored in the decision-making. In a tearful interview, the feeling of loss was still with her six months after admission:

> I had such a nice bungalow and garden. I really enjoyed living there and I have precious memories. If only I could go back.

One resident was resentful toward her family:

> After a life commitment to my children they've dumped me. I did all that work for nothing. I've saved all my life - to come to this. (Mrs Crisp, Elizabeth House)

For others, relief was the main feeling:

> I knew I couldn't live alone, I was so frightened and nervous. I was so relieved when I knew I could come. (Mrs Townsend, The Rectory)

For another couple, the transition was eased following a decision to enter together:

> Although we were managing well at home with a fair level of support, we were also thinking and looking at private homes about a year prior to coming here. It still made leaving our cottage difficult but at least we knew what to expect. (Mr and Mrs Smith, Oaklands)

These statements all reveal residents' attitudes towards leaving 'home' and show how each individual reacted differently to their admission based on experience and expectation.

Some people, such as Mr and Mrs Smith, struggled at home and welcomed the transition into residential care, seeing it as a time of anticipation and planning: for others, like Mrs Grosvenor the loss of home was overwhelming.

Place of residence prior to admission

Table 5.2 shows that residents in both sectors of residential care lived locally prior to admission. However, those who entered local authority homes lived in even closer geographical proximity to the residential home. Thirty-one per cent of local authority residents came from within the catchment area of the parish in which the home was situated but only 16 per cent of those in private homes lived within the same parish boundary as the home.

TABLE 5.2
GEOGRAPHICAL LOCATION OF RESIDENTS PRIOR TO ADMISSION

	Private		Local Authority
	No.	%	%
Same parish	31	16	31
Same social work team	67	33	34
Same social services division	38	19	29
Further distance	64	32	6
	200	100	100

In general, private homes, as well as local authority homes captured a profile of elderly people from the local community: that is, within the boundary of the social services team, but not necessarily in the parish. Unlike the public sector, the private sector also accepted people from further afield.

The flexibility of the private sector to cross geographical boundaries which constrained admissions to public sector homes was highlighted by the fact that 32 per cent entered the private sector from outside social services divisional boundaries, ie they lived in other parts of the county, within the East Anglian region or even outside the United Kingdom. Only 6 per cent of residents crossed the divisional boundary to gain admission to a local authority home. It is interesting to note the two reasons why the private sector attracted residents from outside the County.

1. Potential residents with the means to pay had - in theory - the opportunity to enter any private home, unlike local authority residents they were not constrained by policy decisions based on geography and artificial locational barriers, such as county/divisional boundaries.

2. It was not necessary for home owners to locate their business in central locations or in centres of population. A country retreat was just as attractive to residents and relatives as a central location in the middle of a town. By virtue of their location, therefore, private homes accommodated people from a wider area, as Chapter Three demonstrated.

The analysis of residents' geographical location prior to admission, however, disguised the stepwise mobility that occurred prior to and immediately following retirement with residents moving into Suffolk and within the county itself.

Thirty residents moved into the County in the five years prior to admission before considering a move into residential care. Three moved back to their birthplace following retirement or returned to a place full of happy holiday memories. Others moved to be nearer friends and family:

> I retired from London a few years ago - my friends recommended a bungalow in the area and I moved. (Mrs Jefferys, The Rectory)

> I moved from Kent to live with my daughter when she came to Felixstowe. (Mrs Preece, The Rest)

Others made short distance moves to be closer to family:

> I was previously living in Norwich and then I moved to Debenham five years ago as my husband wanted a larger garden. We were only there one year when he died, so I moved again to be near my daughter. (Mrs Long, Oaklands)

Nineteen people (9 per cent) planned their moves straight into a private home from outside the county. Similarly twenty-six (41 per cent) of the moves from outside the social services divisional boundary were planned from either relatives' homes or other institutional settings. One example is given by Mrs Dove who moved due to inadequate care in another home:

> I was living in a private home in Reigate - it was a voluntary home and it didn't provide night care. I spotted this one in the paper and decided to move. (Mrs Dove, The Dingle)

Composition of residents' households

Table 5.3 shows the composition of the residents' household prior to admission.

TABLE 5.3
COMPOSITION OF RESIDENTS' FORMER HOUSING

	Private		Local Authority
	No.	%	%
Alone	120	60	60
Spouse	28	14	13
Other relative(s)	28	14	17
Friend	4	2	9
Other (institution)	20	10	1
	200	100	100

The majority of people (60 per cent) lived alone and were isolated in terms of household structure. This was particularly true of women going into private residential care (63 per cent). For many, living alone brought difficulties with its associated feelings of loneliness and isolation from the outside world, and was identified as a particular vulnerability point in the journey into residential care.

The psychological feeling of becoming a burden on non-household and family members was difficult for some:

> I was frightened living alone and I knew I was becoming a burden to everyone around. (Mrs West, Oaklands)

For some recently bereft of a partner, living alone became a new and strange experience. An example was provided by Mr Houghton (Greenfields) who:

> never bothered about cooking and cleaning - too late to start at my age. My wife spoilt me and I've not been used to being on my own since.

Mrs Crisp (Elizabeth House) reported:

> When my husband died he took my life with him.

There were also a group of females unique in private care (12 per cent) who lived with non-relatives in other private or local authority homes or long-term psychiatric or geriatric hospitals. This meant that some people had already gone through one process of admission from the community to an institutional setting. One resident, for example, came from a convent because of her senile dementia, inappropriate behaviour in such a setting.

Significant differences were found between men and women in the private sector, not only in terms of those living alone and with 'others' but in respect of those living as husband or wife. A greater percentage (50 per cent) of men lived with their wives prior to admission compared with the 8 per cent of women who lived with their husbands. This confirms the finding in Chapter Four that men who entered residential care were more likely to be married or recently bereft of their wife.

Mr Garrett, featured in Chapter 4, was a typical example of a dependent married man cared for by his wife prior to admission. Although most wives lived nearby and visited daily, institutional life proved a very difficult and lonely experience for some who like the Garretts became separated because of physical frailty. There were fewer married men like this in the local authority sector - possibly because the local authority was less flexible to admit a married couple at the same time or, alternatively, the social worker attempted to keep partners together in the community for as long as possible.

Living with relatives reduced the risk of residential care - only 14 per cent of private sector residents lived with relatives (apart from spouse). However, the purpose behind such a move to live with offspring often reflected the residents' need to be looked after and cared for. The consequent change in the role relationships between family members sometimes proved difficult for all parties, particularly where elderly people felt they had lost part of their security and to some extent their independence.

Such people who lived with relatives were also vulnerable to further moves:

> Mother tried to stir up arguments, so we gave her an ultimatum - live with us or go into a home. She came to live with us but it was difficult and we decided to move her into a home. (Son of Mrs Donnington, Conifers)

Although the minority lived with relatives, family generally lived in close proximity. A number of people moved to the area to be near family and although no questions were asked in the survey about birthplace, the majority of residents lived locally for several years and had family in the vicinity.

Informal sources of support

The levels and sources of informal support which residents received prior to admission reflected their proximity to family networks. Help and support from family and friends was generally available for all but 22 per cent of those who entered the private sector as Table 5.4 illustrates. The largest support came from residents' children (24 per cent).

TABLE 5.4
INFORMAL SUPPORT AT HOME

	Private		Local Authority	
	No.	%	No.	%
Relatives	108	54	91	76
Friends	27	13	17	14
Neighbours	32	16	30	25
Others	34	17	12	10
No support	43	22	17	14
Number of residents=	200		120	

(Some residents received support from more than one source).

The nature of support received from such informal sources ranged from practically-orientated tasks like washing heavy items or a car service to just 'popping in for a chat'. In contrast to these 'neighbourly' tasks, more personal care tasks, eg washing and dressing were carried out mainly by daughters and wives (44 per cent). Some spouses supported husbands with high levels of physical and mental dependency, and went to great lengths to prevent admission. People like Mrs Garrett who struggled to care for her husband, particularly when he suffered bouts of amnesia was such an example. Other wives or husbands struggled to provide some sort of family life while caring for a partner suffering dementia. In some cases neighbours coped with heavy personal tasks. As a social worker expressed:

The neighbour got her up, toiletted her and did domestic chores as well as put her to bed. (Mrs Williams, The Limes)

Although elderly people were well supported by family and neighbours, private sector residents were isolated in terms of their participation in community groups, with low membership or allegiance to any group or society. Few, therefore, took advantage of groups involving elderly people or participated in local social clubs. Their networks hinged around family, neighbours and more formal support systems.

Formal sources of support

The majority of the sample received formal support from statutory services, ie both Health and Social Services. Table 5.5 shows that 63 per cent of those who entered private residential care and 79 per cent of those going into local authority homes received services from one or more agency. Only three people, however, in the private sector received an intense package of community care (that is, more than two services) to enable them to remain at home: for most people this consisted of a home help service. Thirty one per cent of residents took advantage of the service, although the support was for very short periods of time in the week (for example, one or two hours on average). Only 4 per cent already engaged private domiciliary care. On the whole, people did not, therefore, choose private residential care because of past experience of private care while at home.

TABLE 5.5
SERVICES RECEIVED PRIOR TO ADMISSION

	Private		Local Authority	
	No.	%	No.	%
None	75	37	25	21
Home help	63	31	68	57
Meals on wheels	31	15	56	47
District nurse/ health visitor	32	16	23	19
Social worker	21	10	23	19
General Practitioner	19	9	10	8
Day care	18	9	44	37
Private domiciliary care	8	4	2	2
Other	51	25	48	40
Number of residents=	200		120	

(Some residents received support from more than one source)

Apart from service-based resources, few (10 per cent) made regular use of the professional skills of a social worker or GP (9 per cent) during the five years prior to admission. Although need and appropriateness of service were not investigated, and despite the low numbers in receipt of intense formal services, residents in general did not feel inadequately supported.

However, there were a group of ten men (33 per cent of all men) only found in private care and not in local authority care who were not supported in the community and did not receive help from relatives and friends (Table 5.6). Mr Bacton at The Grange was an example of such a man isolated from informal sources of help after the death of his wife. He reported:

> It was okay till my wife died but I had such a poor relationship with my son I just didn't get any support.

TABLE 5.6
INFORMAL SUPPORT TO MEN AT HOME

	Private		Local Authority
	No.	%	%
Support from friends/ relatives etc.	20	67	97
No support	10	33	3
	30	100	100

This is surprising as much of the literature highlights the fact that men living alone tend to receive a greater input of services than women in the same situation. It is an interesting finding as it indicates the presence of a number of independent, professional men, seeking care for reasons other than physical support.

There was also a significant presence in the private sector of a group of women who received no formal support whatsoever and another group of those who lived alone (40 per cent) with significantly less support than similar groups in the local authority sector. This finding is interesting as it supports a commonly held view of people who entered private care and provides evidence of a group of women who entered the private sector not because they were in 'physical need' of care, but because they were lonely, bereft of company and living alone.

Married couples in private residential care were more likely to be mutually supportive and less dependent on help from other relatives and friends than displayed by those who were widowed, single and divorced, who received their main support from offspring.

The evidence also shows that wives and husbands were well supported by social and health services in their attempt to care, with 86 per cent receiving formal support. Such families may have been reluctant to become a burden on sons and daughters and turned in the first instance for help to formal supports.

Although formal services supported married couples in their attempts to retain independence, the same cannot be said for all of those who lived with and were cared for by families. Twelve of the fifteen women who lived with daughters or daughters-in-law received no formal support whatsoever.

This evidence confirms the conclusion of Moroney (1976) that there is a trend among providers of service to establish priorities among potential users. Elderly people who live alone or just with their spouses are more likely to receive services, while those who live with their children or within an extended kin network are more likely to be denied help, particularly if they are female. This supports the argument that the state intervenes when the family cannot continue, with the assumed implication that the family should care.

The extent to which residents felt adequately supported was important despite the level of service they received, and this was reflected in their comments on their ability to manage. Caution must be taken in interpreting such statements, as some residents glorified a less than ideal situation, and in a number of cases, resident and relative perspectives on coping capacity and ability to manage at home differed. One resident, who felt very resentful about her admission, commented:

> I could manage quite well on my own, despite no help from my son. I never thought about giving up as everything was okay. (Mrs Swan, Fairlawns)

Her social worker reported:

> She could manage well on her own. The family just didn't want her.

Adding a different viewpoint to the situation, her son said:

> She was slowly deteriorating - she couldn't cook or look after herself and started doing silly things that old people do.

Such statements of residents' 'coping' abilities reflected relatives' own anxieties and difficulties.

Although a quarter of those who entered private care did not receive any formal help, the majority of people felt well supported: inadequate support was a background factor leading to admission for only 20 per cent of residents.

Reasons for admission

In the five years prior to admission, elderly people interviewed in the study experienced a variety of circumstances and events leaving them vulnerable to entry into residential care (Table 5.7).

TABLE 5.7
BACKGROUND FACTORS TO ADMISSION INTO PRIVATE AND LOCAL AUTHORITY HOMES*

	Private		Local Authority
	No.	%	%
Physical deterioration	130	65	65
Mental deterioration	84	42	49
Accident/sudden illness	62	31	36
Bereavement	54	27	12
Inadequate support	40	20	6
Loneliness	36	18	12
Family unable to care	36	18	20
Family unwilling to care	6	3	9
Pressure from others	14	7	7
Feelings of being a burden	10	5	2
Main carer in care	2	1	6
Other (including general inability to cope, homelessness)	46	23	44
Number of residents=	200		

(Some residents had multiple background factors)

* Within five years of admission

The majority of elderly people entered the private sector with a background of deteriorating health, commonly associated with old age, and fragile networks of support necessary to keep them independent at home. Bereavement of a carer or a spouse was a particular reason for a lack of support. The main reason directly linked to admission was, however, the pressure and influence of other 'operators', generally family, who became increasingly unable to care for their parents and older members of their family (Table 5.8).

TABLE 5.8
SPECIFIC FACTORS LEADING DIRECTLY TO ADMISSION INTO PRIVATE AND LOCAL AUTHORITY HOMES

	Private No.	Private %	Local Authority %
Pressure from other(s)	98	49	50
Family unable to care	42	21	30
Family unwilling to care	10	5	8
Physical deterioration	12	6	12
Mental deterioration	8	4	24
Accident	46	23	15
Inadequate support	20	10	11
Vacancy	44	22	7
Isolation/burden	24	12	11
Temporary/permanent loss of significant other	14	7	11
Number of residents=	200		

(Some residents had multiple background factors)

The four main reasons for entry into residential care were extracted: physical and mental deterioration, pressure from others and family inability to care. Residents were attributed a score according to the number of reasons stated. Few (8 per cent) residents overall experienced all four factors in the process of their admission: the majority - in both sectors - had at least two or more of these factors present (70 per cent of residents in private care and 82 per cent of residents in local authority care stated two or more of the four main reasons for their admission).

All possible combinations were examined. Thirteen per cent of residents who entered private care stated that a deterioration in physical condition linked with pressure from others to seek a residential home placement was the most significant combination.

A similar combination of reasons was found relating to local authority residents, although top of their list was mental deterioration accompanied by an inability of family to continue caring (12 per cent). Reasons for admission among private sector residents are considered first, followed by a comparison of local authority residents.

Physical frailty

Failing health was one of the vulnerability points identified by residents and relatives. The majority of people (65 per cent) who entered residential care suffered a deterioration in their physical health or experienced a sudden illness or accident in the previous five years (Table 5.8). This was a major factor leading to admission for residents irrespective of levels of dependency or confusion. Physical illness was grouped according to the classification used in the Chronically Sick and Disabled Persons Act 1972.

Although overall 20 per cent said they suffered from general frailty over a number of years, the majority of residents mentioned a specific complaint. The main conditions experienced by residents were strokes (12 per cent); arthritis (10 per cent); a sensory impairment (19 per cent) - mainly blindness or hearing problems and heart attacks (6 per cent).

Twenty six people (13 per cent) experienced a variety of physical illnesses in the previous five years: for example, Mr Burton (Eastcliff) who had failing eyesight, poor mobility and repeated bronchial attacks.

Physical decline alone, however, was not a sufficient reason in itself to catapult people into residential care and 83 per cent of residents specified one other factor or series of accompanying factors, which reduced their ability to remain at home and made them vulnerable to residential care.

A fall or an accident was often a consequence of a loss of health and an inability to manage alone. A quarter of those with a background of physical deterioration specified accidents, illness and further physical frailty as a reason directly leading to admission.

Not surprisingly, over half (55 per cent) of the residents found to be dependent or very dependent entered care due to their physical condition and specifically came into a home following an accident or illness. In some instances the process of admission was accelerated, for those suffering from illness, by a move away from home (Table 5.10). For 24 people (12 per cent) an accident at home resulted in a hospital admission, which had many consequences in terms of subsequent moves in the process. Mrs Taylor (The Copse) who lived alone since her husband's death in 1968, fell at home after a heart attack which led to a hospital admission; as a result of the accident she was frightened and lacked confidence to return home and manage alone. Mrs Barford (The Rest) who was frightened of further falls after being discharged from hospital to await a local authority vacancy, immediately took to her bed. In this case, a private sector home with an immediate vacancy provided a ready option for both resident and family who became anxious that a local authority vacancy would never transpire.

Rehabilitation at home, particularly after a stroke or an amputation, proved unsuccessful and unrealistic for others, where a change of environment and physical layout was necessary to accommodate their changed physical conditions. Mrs Stricklands (Fenlands) who, after waiting six months in hospital for such a place to be available, was told by an occupational therapist within hours of moving to a sheltered housing scheme, that the flat chosen would not be suitable for her wheelchair. A list of private homes was offered as an alternative.

For 23 independent elderly people, the experience of a fall or generally not feeling well over a period of time led to a considered decision to enter residential care. Although able to look after themselves, a quarter entered care without a specific reason, just with a fear of further physical deterioration. This was often accompanied by fears of becoming a burden, particularly where a carer was marginally involved. Conditions such as a loss of sight, or experience of a slight stroke brought some to realise their vulnerability and frailty. A decline in ability to self-care and maintain a 'reasonable' standard at home or even a fear of not being able to survive another winter led others to the decision to enter a home, particularly if this decision was reinforced by relatives and professionals.

Being alone, lonely with continuing fears of illness, particularly during the night, were concerns voiced by a majority of the 62 per cent of those who lived alone. There was some justification in their fear because those who lived alone were more vulnerable to accidents and falls than those living with relatives and friends. Nineteen people moved into private care because of the difficulty in managing alone.

A very small but different group of nineteen people in private care were those who chose a private home with a view to providing a period of temporary convalescence after a hospital stay, as a holiday break from the family, or from the isolation they experienced at home. Following a short term stay, four people decided to remain and transferred to the status of permanent residents. Failing health as a consequence of growing older was not significant as a single factor leading to admission. The majority who suffered physical frailty also experienced a number of other circumstances and events of a physical and social kind behind their admission to care.

Mental deterioration as a reason for admission

Eighty four (42 per cent) elderly people who entered private residential care suffered a deterioration in their mental health within a five year period prior to admission. The majority (61 people or 73 per cent of this group) were physically independent but confused. Only 9 per cent of the sample of 200 (18 people) specified continuing mental deterioration alone as a direct and specific factor that led to their entry, which again indicated that admission resulted from a culmination of circumstances.

Three accompanying conditions appeared important:

1. A confused elderly person was vulnerable to residential care if they displayed signs of wandering and/or continued to have a series of accidents. Twenty six per cent of those who suffered mental deterioration specified an accident or an illness as a direct factor of admission. A relative of one resident reported:

> It started off with her burning saucepans and getting more and more confused. The GP, social worker and warden were anxious, but it was only after a series of falls that they would do anything. (Son of Mrs Knight, The Orchard)

2. A lack of support networks also escalated the process of admission. This was mainly due to the family's inability to cope with the level of mental deterioration portrayed by the elderly person (29 per cent) or the death of a carer (6 per cent). This shows that it was not only the presence or absence of support networks that was important but the ability of the network to support the elderly person. Those who suffered a deterioration in their

mental state were more likely to be living with relatives or in homes already (60 per cent) than alone (36 per cent), or with a spouse (41 per cent) which indicates that the inability of relatives and others to cope was an important accompanying factor.

3. Overwhelmingly with a state of confusion, the influence of others was significant in initiating a move from hospital and home to residential care. Fifty one (61 per cent) of those who suffered confusion in the previous five years specifically entered care through the influence of others, particularly psychiatrists, GPs, social workers and relatives. Particular routes taken by confused people into the three specialist homes for elderly mentally infirm people mentioned in Chapter Four, graphically illustrate the three points. All of these homes were similar in accommodating residents who suffered from a mental disorder of one type or another, ranging from advanced senile dementia to 'nerve trouble'. Residents with schizophrenia and with long histories of psychotic illness were also found among this population. Although residents' diagnoses and prognoses were different, they were found in such homes because of the 'inappropriate' behaviour associated with their condition in other settings and the management difficulties which came as a result.

Mrs Ford at Crabfield was admitted following outbursts of aggressive behaviour and physical abuse which the previous private home could only contain by locking its doors. Miss Reynolds at The Suffolk was manipulative and very demanding and left her former home because of this. Very often, domestic situations and relationships at home broke down as a result.

> Mother tried to commit suicide twice. I was really near breaking point. (Daughter of Mrs Howells, Willow House)

The private sector also accommodated people who could be described as being at the 'heavy end' of dependency - that is, those suffering with physical disabilities such as incontinence, stroke victims, as well as dementia of a severe level.

The private home owners of the three specialist homes and their staff catered for and coped with residents in various states of senile dementia which were often exaggerated by a number of psychiatric problems such as a release of sexual inhibitions, or symptoms of personality disorders. For example, some owners reported:

> She always had a pathetic personality, but it really came out when she was with us.

> A ruthless personality greatly exaggerated by the dementia.

> He is so difficult to handle - he has a chest infection and is a stroke victim. He is very sick. Apart from this he's very aggressive and sexually orientated.

All three homes could be described as the 'end of the road' for 44 (22 per cent) residents who had already passed through one system - either hospital

Some residents perceived their relatives' inability to care as their unwillingness to care. Mrs Bowden at Limestone felt very resentful and purposely shunned contact with her daughter:

> I wanted to stay at home, but the children wouldn't help - they should have.

Her daughter said:

> She's always been grudging towards her family - we were just trying to help her.

Where relationships between family members were vulnerable for a number of years prior to admission, a move to live with relatives or friends triggered a potentially volatile situation. Family discord, without the elderly person necessarily being the focus, led two families to withdraw support and place the elderly person in a homeless situation.

It was not only unwilling families who placed elderly people in such vulnerable positions but a small number of private home owners showed signs of their unwillingness to continue caring, particularly if residents displayed signs of aggression and dementia. One instance was recorded where relatives were asked to find an alternative placement within 24 hours.

Bereavement

Bereavement, meaning the permanent loss of a spouse or main carer through death, was a significant background factor for 54 (27 per cent) of those who entered private care.

Temporary loss, through hospitalization or institutionalization, was a less significant factor: only two people (1 per cent) specified it as a reason for admission.

The severe sudden loss experience of bereavement was an important factor for a quarter of the women and 40 per cent of the men who entered care, many of whom were dependent (30 per cent) or confused (23 per cent). In twelve examples, the shock following the bereavement of a husband or wife escalated mental or physical deterioration. For example:

> My husband died suddenly in November. I was soon in hospital with double pneumonia. (Mrs Sticklands, Fenlands)

Where bereavement accompanied physical decline, the bereaved partner was often left without any day-to-day support systems. Four people (7 per cent) found that support from neighbours, friends and even family was temporary and a lack of constant, stable support networks influenced them in considering a move. For example:

> After my husband died, I had to go into hospital as a result of an accident. My neighbours just didn't continue to put in the same level of support they had offered over the years and as a result I couldn't return home. (Mrs Govan, The Limes)

Feelings of loneliness and depression also followed a bereavement to the extent that a few people unsuccessfully attempted to take their own life. Lack of personal care was also symptomatic as one man who was very low and tearful throughout the interview summed up his experience:

> When my wife died, it was killing - she took my whole life with her. (Mr Scott, The Suffolk)

Natural feelings of helplessness and hopelessness after such a loss were expressed. Mrs Gipping, who had been totally devoted to her husband, said:

> I was no good on my own. I was so anxious I don't know what I might have done. (The Limes)

After a short time on her own, Mrs Gipping had a nervous breakdown which resulted in her not eating or sleeping and finally her admission to a psychiatric hospital. She never returned home.

The majority (78 per cent) of residents who came directly into private homes as a result of a bereavement or because their main carer was also in care were, however, physically independent. This suggests that there were other reasons leading to admission. For sixteen (29 per cent of the 54 who were bereft) who were in command of their own situations, moving into a private home was seen as an alternative accommodation solution. Some felt their houses were too big and wanted to make one final step rather than a series of moves at a later time when they might be incapacitated and unable to make such a decision.

One woman had made an agreement with her late husband to enter a home should anything happen to either of them. She had even gone to the extent of choosing and visiting certain homes.

> Previous to my husband's death, we had made pact that neither of us would live alone - we'd had bad experiences in the past caring for our own families. We would go into a home. When the GP also advised us about going in together we took it seriously and started looking. (Mrs Bell, Conifers)

Although entry depended, to some extent, on the vacancy state within a particular home, these cases illustrate the flexibility of the private sector to accommodate an elderly person at their convenience. 18 per cent (10) of those bereaved entered specifically because of the availability of a vacancy.

Vacancy

A minority of people (22 per cent) took the opportunity to enter a private home while there was a vacancy.

Twenty-five people (58 per cent of those taking advantage of such a vacancy) were in the professional classes and were in a position to pay for their placement (Table 4.5). Although some said they were not in 'need' of care at all, the residential care resource was accessible to them because they could afford it. They entered less through 'need' than a variety of other reasons.

Pressure and the influence of others

> 'She can't cope ... something must be done'.

A considerable section in the gerontological literature notes the relationship between choice and control held by elderly people and the 'success' of their admission into residential care (Willcocks et al, 1987). Elderly people who were consulted on their choice of home and timing of admission were found to be more settled once in a home than those who did not anticipate and direct their route into residential care (Tobin & Lieberman, 1976). One of the advantages put forward for the growth of private care has been the control and choice it offers elderly people in their admission to care (Wade et al, 1983; Weaver et al, 1985a). However, other research points to the fact that the idea of a referral for residential care often begins with someone else (Townsend, 1962; ADSS, 1985).

This study looked at the pressure and influence of other people in the move to residential care and the extent to which people finally resided in their choice of home. The latter is covered in following chapters. This section looks at the source and nature of pressure and circumstances under which elderly people were influenced. Half of all elderly people interviewed felt they were influenced, persuaded or pressurized into a decision about admission to a private home. The pressures were from a number of sources.

Sources of influence and pressure. The main source of pressure was from offspring. Forty one people (42 per cent of those experiencing pressure as a direct factor) said they felt pressurized by their son(s) and/or daughter(s) to enter residential care. Some perceived the anxiety of daughters, in particular, as a pressure factor. An example was provided by Mrs Selway whose only difficulty was her big and dilapidated house:

> My daughter didn't like my being on my own. I could have managed - it was just my daughter's influence and anxiety. (Mrs Selway, The Copse)

The opinions of other family members carried weight in the decision-making process. Mrs Cross (Inglenook) moved from a nursing home to a private residential home because her niece thought she was too institutionalized.
Mrs Cross's niece said:

> I didn't like her being institutionalized on the geriatric ward and after one year I felt she was well enough to move. We wanted her where we could visit. She didn't really need nursing care or a private home but that's where we brought her.

Professional pressure, particularly a GP's or hospital doctor's opinion, carried a great deal of sway with elderly people and their relatives. One resident reported:

> The GP frightened me so much I thought I'd better do something about it. (Mrs Tetley, The Suffolk)

Residents who came via hospital routes experienced pressure from doctors to 'clear the beds'.

> I went to Ipswich Hospital and then to convalesce at Felixstowe. The doctor wanted me out quickly - it was that bad weather at the time (snow) and I couldn't be on my own so I came here. (Mrs Bates, Limestone)

No GP followed up with arrangements for admission in any of these examples.

In a number of instances just a statement such as 'she can't cope at home' added to the anxieties of relatives and residents. This became a powerful trigger in the journey into residential care, often reinforcing relatives' views of the situation and undermining elderly people's self-confidence about managing at home.

In two instances, relatives were asked to look for a private home by hospital consultants; in one private home (The Suffolk) pressure was put on patients - by the home manager and a ward sister - to accept the ready option of a private home placement.

Pressure was also exerted in a more direct fashion by others with compulsory powers to remove elderly people from their home (either through environmental or mental health acts).

The housing department was involved in closing tenure on one lady. For another, the environmental health officer threatened eviction under Section 47 of the Public Health Act 1936 after she was found in 'pools of urine, squalor and filth'. This lady had little choice. Ten others who were in hospital felt social workers and other professionals 'behind the scenes' were taking decisions out of their hands.

What other reasons fuelled anxiety and reinforced the view that the elderly person could not cope?

Elderly people, vulnerable through loss or lack of support, following a bereavement felt the decision was taken out of their hands (32 per cent of people under pressure had experienced a bereavement). It was not surprising that people going through a bereavement felt helpless in the immediate period after their loss. For a number the significance of making a decision to move into residential care was not apparent until they had actually moved home.

Pressure from other sources was particularly evident if an element of physical or mental deterioration together with a series of accidents was involved.

The journey into local authority care

The reasons surrounding admission to private residential care were reviewed in the light of admission to the local authority residential sector. Although there were a number of similarities in both the reasons and journey into care, this section only examines the significant differences between the two sectors and describes the differences in the process of admission into local authority homes.

Deterioration in mental state

One of the major differences between the two sectors was the level of confusion found among residents (Table 4.13) and as a result, one of the main reasons for admission of elderly people to local authority residential care was a deterioration in their mental state (49 per cent). Not only were there greater numbers of confused people in local authority care, but in comparison with a similar profile of people entering private care, there were different circumstances surrounding their process of admission, eg people with mental deterioration in the private sector entered because of their family's inability to continue in a caring role.

Twenty five (21 per cent) residents also specified a physical deterioration in health as an accompanying reason for entry: this figure compares to 9 per cent in the private sector. This finding confirms one of the conclusions reached in Chapter Four - that is the local authority sector was involved in caring for a group of people who were confused and physically frail.

A number of confused elderly people (51) prior to coming into local authority care lived alone and received support not from friends or family but from local authority services (Table 5.5). A greater percentage of people in local authority care received services such as meals-on-wheels (47 per cent : 15 per cent) and day care (37 per cent : 9 per cent).

Confused people who ended up in this sector, therefore, were kept 'independent' until their level of confusion reached a point where life at home was unsupportable by formal or informal sources. Eighteen families of elderly people in local authority care said that their difficulty in coping with the mental condition of elderly relatives, despite the support of such services, specifically led them to seek a private residential home before they broke down under the strain.

Mrs Jinks (Richey House) graphically illustrates this point. As a result of her increasing confusional and paranoid states, she moved to live with her son and daughter-in-law. The family found it difficult to cope, despite regular short-term stays at a local authority home. Increasing pressure on the family and on the son's marriage forced Mrs Jinks' daughter-in-law to telephone social services to demand that a home be found for the old lady. However, during the social work visit that followed, the offer of a residential placement was turned down in preference to additional support. Mrs Jinks' daughter-in-law said:

> I felt so guilty, even just wanting to put her name on the list.

Although the social worker felt she was not coping, the daughter-in- law agreed to continue in her caring role with extra support. The situation lasted a couple of months when the strain of caring led to serious and violent marital difficulties between the son and his wife. As a result, Mrs Jinks was eventually admitted to a local authority home.

Why were more confused elderly people entering local authority care?

In addition to similar groups of confused residents in private homes, the local authority accommodated confused people with additional handicaps not generally found in the private sector. The local authority was more likely to accommodate those residents who were 'undesirable'. A number of people described as such, because of their self-neglect, squalid living conditions or bizarre life style, tended to be confused.

1. There were more examples in this sector of people living in squalor, alone or isolated to the outside world. The majority of these people had no other advocates and in most cases, were only discovered by formal service agencies after a crisis or a string of complaints from neighbours.

2. A number of residents in this sector were highly vulnerable because of their confused state and entered a home via guardianship - with the local authority acting as guardian. With the local authority holding responsibility it was more likely to provide its own accommodation to contain these residents in care.

Mrs Hillfield suffered intermittent confusional states with paranoid delusions: she had been on medication all her life and spent several years moving in and out of hospital; she was also confused. All attempts to admit Mrs Hillfield to hospital or a local authority home failed despite the involvement of several agencies.

A private placement was found by her son and niece who took the situation out of the hands of the social worker. However, Mrs Hillfield refused to stay and returned home. Although attempts were made to support her, the crisis came when she was locked out of doors. On the arrival of the GP and social worker she refused all medication and any voluntary attempt at a hospital admission. Mrs Hillfield was finally admitted under Section 3 of the Mental Health Act 1983, which was transferred to guardianship following a stabilisation of her mental condition.

3. A number of confused people were already in the local authority system. Some people admitted to hospital on a short-term basis 'floated' around the system until a bed in a suitable local authority home became available: that is, they often went from one hospital to another before being placed.

Residents described as 'management problems' in particular were often moved around the system.

In many cases the wait for a local authority vacancy was long, particularly if the elderly person was not in an 'at risk' situation by virtue of being in hospital. It was not unusual to find people in the public sector who had already been in two or three hospitals prior to admission. One lady found herself waiting over a year in a local cottage hospital for a vacancy in a local authority home.

Sequence of care: source of admission

The evidence in Table 5.9 shows that a large group of people entered both sectors directly from their home in the community. Admissions from hospitals were also prominent particularly in the public sector.

TABLE 5.9
SOURCE OF ADMISSION

	Private		Local Authority
	No.	%	%
Own home	82	41	41
Hospital	71	35	48
Other (institution/ relatives)	47	24	11
	200	100	100

The route into private care from 'home'

The evidence suggested that people from this source were supported informally in order to remain in the community, particularly by a spouse or other relative with whom they lived. Half of this group also received formal services and as expected they tended to be more independent than those who entered from hospital.

A very similar pattern emerged for those who entered the public sector, although there were no differences in dependency according to the route followed. These people, too, (32 per cent) were often supported by relatives who were reaching a breaking point in their ability to care. For example, Mrs Lee at Eastcliffe said:

> I just couldn't do for myself; even my home help found it too much to cope with me. I became too dependent on my family (home help). I can see that now.

The hospital route

The evidence suggested that hospitalization precipitated admission of certain groups, particularly vulnerable elderly people living alone or people who lacked an adequate support network of friends and family to which they could return.

Forty eight people, 68 per cent, of those coming through a hospital system into private care lived alone and were unsupported at home by formal services. Those who lived with and were supported by non-family members, such as friends, or were in other institutional settings, were also more likely to enter private care via the hospital route. [64 per cent of those supported by 'others' came via hospital; 7 per cent from home.]

This indicated that the presence of a stable and reliable support system was vital if people were to return home from hospital. Some elderly people who lived in a private home or with 'others' could not be guaranteed a return to the same setting as often an admission to hospital was a turning point at which carers withdrew their support, forcing elderly people to search for alternative accommodation. Mrs Jackson (The Conifers), for example, was admitted from sheltered housing suffering from anorexia but was unable to return because the warden would not allow her back.

Of the confused residents in the private sector, 34 (38 per cent of 90) entered from a local psychiatric hospital setting. It was people like Miss Reynolds (The Suffolk) who were classed as 'too good' to require long-term hospital care, but were unable to live and cope at home. Similar people entered local authority homes from hospital. However, three people - although physically independent - suffered from senile dementia or a psychiatric illness and were in general long-term psychiatric or geriatric wards which were scheduled for closure. A return to their families in the community was unrealistic, particularly where networks had been severed years before entry to hospital. They were just waiting for a move to one home or another.

The nature of admission

Private sector admission

The majority of admissions into residential care were planned as Table 5.10 illustrates.

TABLE 5.10
THE NATURE OF ADMISSION

	Private		Local Authority
	No.	%	%
Crisis admission	66	33	24
Planned admission	128	64	76
Unknown	6	3	-
	200	100	100

> When he was near discharge we went for a home visit - it was so difficult to arrange the maximum support he needed. When the time came to go back home he threw a wobbly and felt he couldn't go. I got him straight into a private home. (social worker for Mr Tate, Seaview)

TABLE 5.11
SOURCE AND NATURE OF ADMISSION

	Hospital		Home		Other		All	
	No.	%	No.	%	No.	%	No.	%
Private - crisis	31	46	18	27	17	27	66	33
planned	39	31	64	50	24	19	128	64
	70		82		42		194*	
Local - crisis	4	14	20	69	5	17	29	24
authority planned	53	58	30	33	8	9	91	76
	57		50		13		120	

*** six cases unknown**

Mrs Esterene, who was physically frail when admitted to hospital, felt pressurized when the houseman said she needed 24-hour care and wouldn't allow her to return home. A relative said 'We had to look for somewhere pretty quick'. This suggests that once people were ready to leave hospital and were fit enough to go back into a community setting but not able to return home and if there were relatives involved in the decision-making process, then a move into residential care was encouraged. Private residential care proved

Many people who came into the private sector as a result of a crisis were physically frail or suffered a deterioration in their mental state. A fall was regarded as the 'last straw' for 56 (85 per cent) of this group.

Insecurity of tenure was an important factor precipitating a crisis admission. Six people (50 per cent) of those in private rented accommodation arrived in private homes as crisis admissions, reflecting the vulnerable position they were in through lack of ownership. Mr North said:

> I was knocked down by a car and had to go into hospital. My son wanted me to go into a home and I had to because my landlord didn't want me back.

Twenty of the 29 crisis admissions (69 per cent) into local authority care came from home and involved people who were suddenly left bereft of their source of support. They typically found themselves in a situation similar to Mrs Gates (Condor House), who was severely handicapped with multiple sclerosis which confined her to a wheelchair:

> I was alone after my husband died. Four months prior to admission I learnt I had multiple sclerosis and I was deteriorating rapidly. I had to go somewhere. I couldn't cope after his death.

Conclusion

1. This chapter concentrated its attention on the reasons for admission into private and local authority residential care. It demonstrated that no single factor was unique in admission to either sector - elderly people entered residential care for a series of complex reasons which often involved other people. It was often an accumulation of circumstances, both of a physical or mental and social nature that triggered (or led to) an admission into care. The majority of residents in private residential care entered because of physical frailty and an inability of their support networks to sustain them at home any longer. These factors were not unique to residents in the private sector.

2. The extent of overlap in the characteristics of residents in the private and public sectors was considerable; so too there were similarities in the routes followed into care and reasons for seeking such an admission. Not only were there different welfare sectors and systems competing for similar residents (Chapter Four) but access to private and public sectors was along similar lines for the majority of residents.

3. Despite the similarity there were identifiable groups found in one sector or the other. There were a small group of independent people, mainly women, in the private sector who entered because they were lonely, in a number of cases after the death of their husband, and who feared the future alone. For such people a vacancy in a private home provided the opportunity and the ability to pay allowed them access. Another group of women found predominantly in the private sector came from other private homes or long-stay wards in hospitals.

The local authority sector of homes accommodated larger numbers of elderly people who entered because of increasing mental frailty. It also contained a group of 'undesirable' elderly people who may not have had access to private care because of their chaotic living conditions. Such groups entered care either because of a breakdown in their support systems or because they had no support system or advocate.

It is interesting to note that people who entered private care did so because their main carers - families - were unable to care for their physical needs, whereas those who went into local authority homes were admitted after a break in the ability of family to care for the elderly person's mental frailty.

It was only in the three specialist private homes that there were any comparable numbers of confused elderly people to those found in local authority homes. This suggests that home owners, feeling more comfortable with a resident requiring physical care, discouraged those elderly people with confusion from entry.

The three main areas where differences were found between the two sectors were in terms of social class, ownership (Chapter Four) and confusion. There were also differences in the numbers of people in each sector receiving formal support. These three were grouped together with similar variables (see Diagram 5.1) and were accumulated to give an overall indication of the differences in the populations of the 2 sectors. Diagram 5.1 illustrates the considerable overlap between the sectors that resulted from this analysis.

DIAGRAM 5.1
THE EXTENT OF OVERLAP BETWEEN PRIVATE AND PUBLIC SECTORS

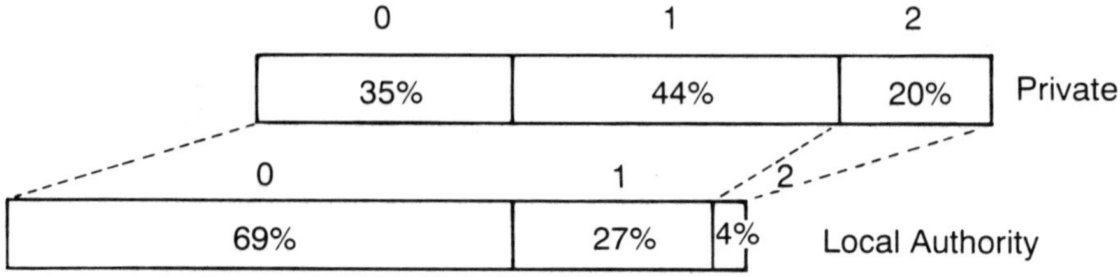

$\chi^2 = 36.302$ df=2 $p < 0.001$

Social Class /

Housing

KEY

0 = % in rented accommodation and manual work

1 = one from each group (0 or 2)

2 = % owner-occupiers professional/ managerial

Physical /

Mental

Dependency

0 = % physically dependent/ mentally confused

1 = one from each group (0 or 2)

2 = % independent/ not confused.

NB *Figures are rounded*

% = percentage of residents

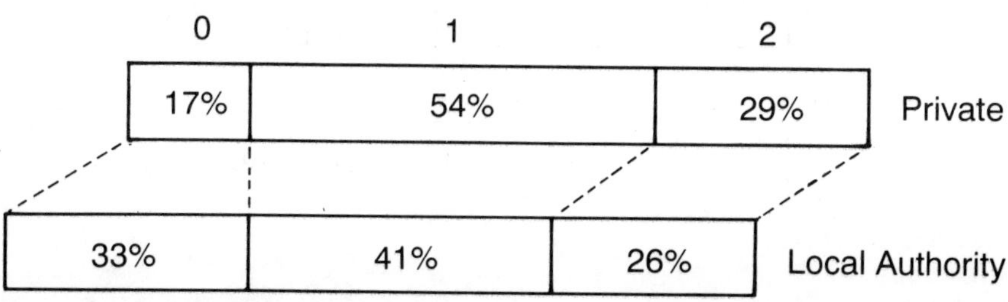

$\chi^2 = 11.573$ df=2 p,0.01

SUPPORT NETWORKS
(formal & informal)

KEY

0 = % receiving informal (1) and formal support (2)

1 = one from each group (i.e. o1 + 21 or o2 + 21 etc)

2 = no support

NB *Figures are rounded*

% = percentage of residents

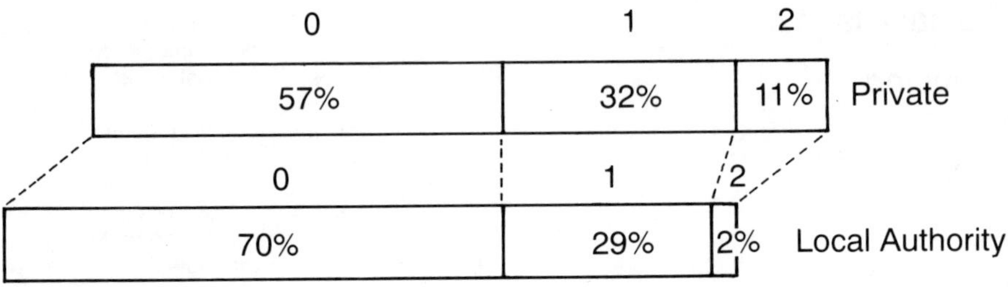

$\chi^2 = 10.927$ df=2 $p<0.01$

TOTAL 1-6 = possible range of scores

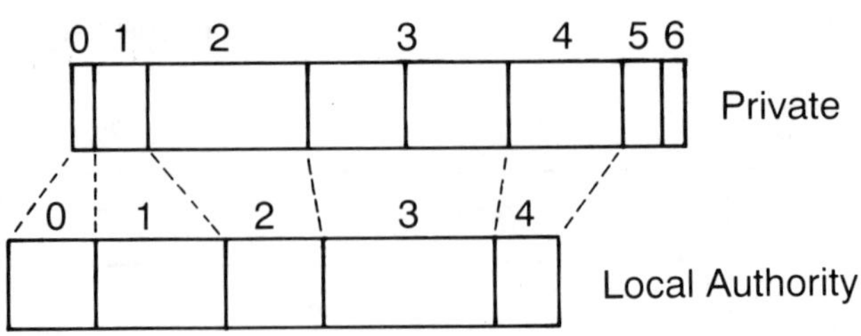

The similarities outweighed the differences.

The greater differences were found among the variables indicating social status and ownership, again reflecting that admission to the private sector hinged upon the ability to pay. Private residential care allowed greater access to those wealthier elderly people who could pay for such care.

4. The ability to pay gave some elderly people access to the network of private homes and provided some indication of why elderly people chose the private sector and why others were restricted and barred from admission. However, Chapter Five also provided a variety of other indications as to why elderly people and their families chose private sector care. An attractive feature of this sector was its flexibility to accommodate people from a wide catchment area, at a time to suit their convenience.

A clear advantage over the local authority sector was the private sector's ability to take people from any geographical location - even from outside the United Kingdom. Although very few elderly people came from abroad in practice, and the majority of residents lived in the locality prior to admission, geographical flexibility was certainly a marketable feature of the sector (Diagram 2.3). With greater mobility of offspring, elderly people have a greater opportunity to end their days in a care setting nearer their children than they might otherwise have had if the private sector had not expanded its provision.

Suffolk is not only a county within commuting distance to London, but also provides an attractive retirement setting for these commuters who want their parents close at hand. The private residential sector has great potential in this area of the country.

5. The private sector was also flexible in that it allowed elderly people and their families to choose when they wanted to enter. Many families, realising they were unable to continue supporting parents or aunts and uncles at home, were able to look around, choose a private home and arrange for admission when it suited all parties.

For many residents in local authority homes there had been an attempt to prevent an admission by the input of formal services such as home help and meals on wheels. Although residents of neither sector had prolonged contact with social workers while at home, those in the local authority sector had already come into contact with the local authority via domiciliary services such as home help organisers, occupational therapists and physiotherapists, who in a number of cases supported an elderly person to remain in the community long after the family felt able and after informal supports were beginning to crack. In this sector, then, it was the professional - a social worker in most cases - that planned the timing of entry.

The situation in the private sector also seemed to be more adaptable to take residents who wanted to transfer from a short to a long-stay. The private sector system also allowed elderly people to gain admission from hospital much quicker than the local authority process where a number of elderly people floated around the system, moving from one hospital to another until a suitable vacancy arose. It was also flexible to take elderly people who had got stuck in the hospital system and who because of their low risk status, were not priority candidates for a bed in a local authority home.

6. A clear thread running throughout this chapter has been the important presence of relatives - not only as support networks but as key influential people in the process of admission. Sons and daughters tended to live in close proximity to their parents and were able to provide a considerable and vital level of support. It was not surprising then that when such support broke down there was a need for elderly people to turn to alternative support. This finding supports other earlier research evidence such as Harbert (1980).

Few elderly people, however, had previous experience of private support systems. It would not have been surprising if a number of elderly people going into private residential care did so because they were satisfied and happy with private domiciliary care. This, however, was not the case. Neither did this group receive high levels of local authority services. Their main supports were informal and from family, friends and neighbours.

With the breakdown in ability to care, relatives took the initiative and sought residential care - in the majority of cases influencing or 'pressurizing' their elderly relative in their future direction of care.

7. Private residential care was not just meeting a housing or accommodation need. Most elderly people sought a setting offering care to meet their physical and mental health needs. Among the various reasons for admission, the feeling of frailty and subsequent need for physical care and attention was expressed by most new residents. A 'secure' caring environment was attractive to many in the sample who suffered regular falls and occasional accidents. The majority of residents also looked at provision that replicated some of the tending aspect that had previously been provided at home by their family. Families also saw home owners and their staff taking over the day-to-day responsibility for the elderly person's physical well-being.

Only a small minority of residents chose private residential care to satisfy an accommodation need only. These residents were generally women, who being independent, were able to take their time to select between a variety of options and choose the accommodation most suitable within their price range. They viewed their private residential home as a hotel setting providing privacy and independence.

8. If similar elderly people entered public and private residential care because of similar reasons, what made some people choose private care while others opted for a public care provision? Chapter Five touched on some of the answers to this question, but Chapter Six explores this further and looks at whether residential care was inevitable, what alternatives were available and how many people chose one sector or the other.

6 Private residential care: preference or pragmatic choice?

Private residential care: preference or pragmatic choice?

The majority of elderly people in the study were vulnerable to residential care because of a number of circumstances which eventually led to their admission into a private home. Many residents were physically frail or mentally dependent in one way or another and were supported by relatives and professionals who were anxious about their ability to live independently. Through such anxiety, pressure was directed at elderly people to apply for residential care. Chapter Five also showed that a similar population in the same way, entered local authority care. The question remains therefore as to why some people entered private homes while others, facing the same events and circumstances, eventually entered homes provided by the local authority.

Chapter Six attempts to answer a series of related questions which are central to policy makers and planners of residential provision.

1. Was residential care inevitable for those groups of elderly people with broadly similar characteristics and in similar circumstances, described in the two previous chapters?

2. Were there particular people for whom residential care was inevitable?

3. Under what circumstances was residential care inevitable?

4. Were people exercising a positive choice for residential care?

5. Were prospective residents consciously making decisions between public and private residential care? Did people enter private residential care through preference or were they excluded from alternative residential provision, for example voluntary or local authority sectors of care, and vice versa?

6. Who were the people who expressed a preference for the private sector and under what circumstances could they exercise such a preference?

It will be shown that many residents in both sectors of care had no option but to enter a home. Few people who entered private care had alternatives open to them in the community; where choice existed it was between different residential settings in the private sector. For the majority in both public and private sectors, there were no community alternatives available, with the result that residential care appeared to be inevitable.

It became clear that many residents felt compelled to seek placements in private residential homes because they thought there was a scarcity of places in the public sector: among private home residents,only a minority (10 per cent) indicated that they would have spurned a place in local authority accommodation. From this it could be shown that those entering the private sector felt deprived of the opportunity to opt for a public sector place.

In those instances where it appeared the residents had a 'choice', the decision was often determined by the availability of an appropriate place at the crucial time: hence it was effectively a pragmatic choice. An appropriate place was a home in an attractive and familiar neighbourhood; one which offered privacy, security, an emphasis on individuality and which accommodated similar kinds of people.

This chapter looks at the options available to private sector residents and examines how available these alternatives were to them, according to their gender, age, marital status, physical and mental dependency and other circumstances. Alternatives open to local authority residents are highlighted in comparison.

These findings are reviewed in terms of the residential versus community care debate, with a particular focus on the choice between public and private care. In conclusion, the notion of choice within a market model of welfare is discussed in light of the evidence presented.

Methodology and analysis

Three different viewpoints were used to look at the alternatives to private residential care - those of the elderly person, their relative and a professional involved in the process of admission.

Both elderly people and their relatives were asked: "Were there any other options you could have taken other than coming here?" In addition, an open-ended question was introduced asking why other options were not followed.

Although three perspectives were analysed, this chapter is concerned with the residents' view of the alternatives available to them. It looks at the consumer perspective of alternatives and not at the appropriateness of such alternatives or at how realistic they were for each individual. Following initial analysis of the options available to each elderly person the data was recoded as follows:

1. Community care	-	consisted of services which supported an individual living with relatives or friends, remaining at home, or returning to a domestic setting from hospital or other institutional setting (i.e. living in a setting other than an institution).
2. Residential care (private)	-	care provided by an institutional setting
3. Residential care	-	(either private or local authority)
4. Residential (other)	-	care provided in hospital, nursing home or hotel
Residential (both)	-	residents who had the option of both private and public sector homes
5. Residential and Community	-	those with a combination of residential and community care alternatives
(private)	-	only within the private sector of care
(public)	-	only within the public sector of care
(both)	-	both within the private and public sectors of care and other provision

Was residential care inevitable?

Table 6.1 shows that the largest single group in both sectors said that they had no other option than to enter residential care. Significant differences, however, existed between the two sectors in that people in private residential care had more alternatives open to them than those residents in local authority residential provision (58 per cent compared with 41 per cent). In the private sector, one third had options within the residential sector alone.

TABLE 6.1
ALTERNATIVES AVAILABLE TO PRIVATE AND PUBLIC SECTOR RESIDENTS

	Private No.	Private %	Local Authority No.	Local Authority %
1. No alternatives available	84	42	70	59
2. Residential alternatives:				
same sector	44	22	8	7
other sector	10	5	11	9
both sectors/other residential	13	7	14	11
3. Community	28	14	9	7
4. Residential and community:				
same sector	9	4	4	3
other sector	6	3	2	2
both sectors/other residential	6	3	2	2
	200	100	120	100

TABLE 6.2
OPTIONS WITHIN RESIDENTIAL CARE

	Private No.	Private %	Local Authority No.	Local Authority %
*Residential:				
Same sector	53	26	12	10
other sector	16	8	13	11
both sectors/other residential	19	10	16	13
	88	44	41	34

* This Table includes those residents with one other residential option amalgamated with those with both residential and community options (2 and 4 in Table 6.1)

Residential care options

Residential care was inevitable for three-quarters (76 per cent) of those entering private residential care. However, in comparison 86 per cent of local authority residents had no option to consider other than residential care (Table 6.1).

Significant differences existed between the two sectors in terms of available residential provision. Table 6.2 breaks down the figures presented in Table 6.1 to show that a greater percentage of residents in private homes had options *within* the private sector. Few residents in the private sector (18 per cent) pursued alternatives among public sector homes.

In contrast, public sector residents had fewer options within their own sector - few had the choice of another local authority residential home, but more had the choice of a private home. Residential care was, therefore, inevitable for the two groups, but there were more alternatives open to private sector residents, allowing them choice between a selection of private homes.

Community care options

Only a quarter of private sector residents and 14 per cent (an eighth) of those in local authority residential homes felt that they had the opportunity to follow community care options (Table 6.1) - in other words, the opportunity of living with a relative or friend, staying at home or returning to a domestic setting from hospital. This was interesting in view of the fact that elderly people are known to prefer to remain at home rather than enter a home (Sinclair, 1988) and in the light of the resources employed by several agencies to make community care a reality. Whether such alternatives were rejected by potential residents or whether community care was unrealistic for these people is discussed later in this chapter.

The majority of people in the study did not have a choice between various residential and community based options. Only 10 per cent (21) of people in private residential care felt they had the choice of remaining in their community and the choice of different residential homes.

Community care was an option available to few, irrespective of their characteristics, including their mental and physical state. Even ability to pay as a single factor did not necessarily increase the elderly person's chance of having greater options within the community.

Were there any particular circumstances under which residential care was inevitable? Were people, faced by particular circumstances, excluded from any options?

1. Support networks. Living alone, with a spouse or other person did not have any effect on the options available, neither did the nature of informal or formal support have any bearing on the outcome. No differences were found between those who received formal services and those who managed independently at home without a home help, meals on wheels, district nurse, health visitor or social worker.

Residential care was viewed as inevitable despite the nature and extent of support given by various agencies in their attempt to keep elderly people at home for as long as possible.

2. Other significant people in the process. The choice between remaining in the community or entering a home differed depending on who was involved in the admission. Significant 'others' (identified by the elderly people) in the process of admission itself, were influential in opening up or closing off choice for the elderly person. The small group of residents going into private

residential care unaided, had the option of remaining or returning to the community. These were not necessarily independent or lucid. Residential care was more inevitable if the elderly person journeyed through the process with the help of family, professionals or others. This suggests, therefore, that relatives and, in particular, significant others were extremely influential in the elderly person's ultimate decision to enter a home.

TABLE 6.3
SIGNIFICANT 'OTHERS' INVOLVED IN THE PROCESS OF ADMISSION AND OPTIONS AVAILABLE TO PRIVATE SECTOR RESIDENTS

	Family %	Professional %	Other %	None %	All %
None	41	46	39	23	84
Residential:					
private					44
local authority	35	33	48	23	10
other/both					13
Community:	9	10	12	41	28
Residential and community:					
private					9
local authority	8	10	-	-	6
other/both					6
Not known	7	1	1	13	22
	100	100	100	100	200
n =	120	102	32	22	

About half the sample population irrespective of their reasons for admission had no alternatives open to them.

3. Source of admission. Elderly people who entered private residential care from their own homes (or 'other' sources) had more alternatives open to them than those admitted from hospital.

Over half of those coming from hospital were restricted in choice and for the remainder, other options were predominantly concentrated in residential care. Table 6.4 shows the inevitability of moving to a residential setting, faced by people in hospital. Once in hospital there was very little chance or choice of returning home.

TABLE 6.4
SOURCE OF ADMISSION AND OPTIONS AVAILABLE IN THE PRIVATE SECTOR

	Hospital		Other (inc own home)	
	No.	%	No.	%
None	38	54	45	35
Residential and community options	33	46	84	65
	71	100	129	100

This section showed that residential care was unavoidable. Nearly half the residents in the private sector had no alternative but to enter the home they were in at the time of the study. This was particularly true for those elderly people who entered care from hospital with the help of relatives. For the majority of other residents, residential care - predominantly in the private sector - was the only perceived alternative.

Was residential care as inevitable for similar sections of residents in public sector homes?

In all circumstances residential care was more inevitable for local authority residents as already described. Even those people with support enabling them to live at home, those who entered from home rather than hospital and those who planned their future direction of care were less likely to have alternatives open to them than similar residents in the private residential sector.

One explanation for the inevitability of residential care lies in the fact that it was necessary for a professional to be involved in the process of admission to a local authority home. For those who entered local authority care, need for residential care was assessed by a social worker in relation to the available community care alternatives. If community care was a realistic option for local authority residents, then following a professional assessment, residential care would not be followed through. Community care was not often realistic in the professionals' eyes.

Unlike the public sector, no professional assessment of need had to be established as a condition for entry into the private sector. Private sector residents and their relatives were able to determine their own future direction of care. The research showed that relatives could help elderly people with their decision to enter and choice of a residential home unlike in the public sector where relatives and elderly people had to follow a professional judgement of the situation. In the private sector they could decide themselves on their need for residential care and could ignore any feasible package of community care put together by a social worker, viewing it as an undesirable alternative. Residents and relatives in private care, could to a greater extent choose what they wanted. Whereas professional social workers had greater influence in public sector care, relatives had greater influence in private care.

A choice for residential care

The chapter has, so far, highlighted that the majority of residents in the private sector had few community care options but had a variety of other options which were concentrated in the private residential sector.

Twenty four per cent of residents had the option to remain at home (Table 6.1). Why did these people end up in residential care? Were these people exercising a positive choice for residential care instead of community care? Does this mean that a number of people entered residential care out of preference rather than through circumstance? To answer these questions the qualitative data relating to all admissions are explored (Table 6.5).

TABLE 6.5
WHY COMMUNITY CARE/LIVING AT HOME WAS NOT FOLLOWED AS AN ALTERNATIVE TO PRIVATE RESIDENTIAL CARE

	Reason	No.
1.	A positive choice for residential care	29
2.	Relative/professional defines the elderly person as being unable to cope at home	25
3.	Resident felt inadequately or inappropriately supported	21
4.	Residential care as a housing solution	14
5.	Inadequate information	11
6.	Other	50
7.	Not known	50
		200

Although they had the opportunity of remaining in the community, there were a small number of elderly people (29) who made a positive choice to enter private residential care.

For 25 residents it was a professional decision that defined their inability to remain at home or the assessment of relatives that they would be unable to cope in the community and needed residential care.

The ability to remain at home depended in part on how well supported elderly people felt they were. Twenty one people (10 per cent) expressed their dissatisfaction with available domiciliary support, a factor which led them to seek residential care.

For a further 14, admission to residential care was a solution to a housing problem - they were either homeless or living in 'unsatisfactory' accommodation.

1. Residents making a positive choice for residential care

One of the advantages of the private sector is its flexibility and lack of bureaucratic and professional hurdles to gain entry. Elderly people themselves can define their 'coping capacity' in the community, without a professional being involved in defining their need for residential care. If the elderly person did not wish to stay in the community then she could opt to enter a private home provided she had the means to do so. Twenty nine people who could have remained at home chose not to do so but decided instead to enter private residential care.

A number of reasons were given for making this decision. Some people said they could not continue to cope at home through loneliness, following a bereavement or through fear of isolation. Their motivation to maintain an independent life in the community was low and residential care was sought as a solution. A variety of other reasons were given:

> Coming into a home seemed easier than anything else. (Mrs Jones/Fairlawns)

> I could have kept to myself, but I didn't want to be isolated. (Mrs Bolt/Fenlands)

> I just wanted to be waited on. (Mr Brickley/Brookside)

> I didn't look at a home help etc. as I panicked and felt the only solution was a home. (Mrs Drake/The Orchard)

> I didn't want a home help as I knew I'd have to come in here ... one day. I'm too independent and I wanted to do things my own way. (Miss Apricot/The Lawns)

> I didn't even need a home help I was so fit, but I was adamant I wanted to move into a small residential home. (Mrs Hubbard/Conifers)

> I wanted a hotel where I could get complete rest and treatment for my ulcers. (Miss Jones/Fenland)

According to the assessment of relatives, the elderly people described above were not in need of residential care. People were able to define their own need to be looked after and were allowed to express that felt need in the private sector through their ability to pay. To deprive people of their preferred choice would be to enforce their independence in the community.

The majority of people who made a positive choice for residential care were able to do so by their own sources of funding. Twenty five elderly people acted like true consumers because they bought into private care through their own financial means and viewed the transaction between themselves and the home owner similar to that of a guest and hotel manager. Only 4 of the 29 who choose residential care out of preference were in receipt of DHSS funding. The DHSS was not, therefore, providing money for people who by the assessment of the residents or their relatives were defined as 'not in need of residential care'.

Such people who exercised preferences would probably be excluded from the public sector by their failure to demonstrate a need for residential care to a professional social worker.

For a small number (6), the lack of motivation to remain at home led to a break down in their support system. Community care 'packages' were unrealistic as an option if they were not supported by - and acceptable to - elderly people themselves. This supports earlier evidence that even for elderly people receiving support, residential care was no less inevitable if they did not wish to remain at home.

> No other options were presented - I would have refused them anyway. (Mrs Bolt/Fenlands)

2. *A relative or professional definition that the elderly person was unable to cope at home*

Professionals and relatives said that based on a professional assessment 12 per cent of those who entered the private sector were unable to continue living independently at home. This appears a relatively low percentage in light of the fact that half the sample felt pressurized by their offspring to enter a home.

In some instances, it was the general practitioner who was the significant influence in initiating the process by refusing to allow people to return home after a hospital stay because of their inability to cope. For example:

> The GP said I couldn't go back, particularly after I didn't manage very well on the days trial, but I'd love to go back. (Mr Portage, Easton Lodge)

> Conditions at home were unsuitable. Although she was physically capable of looking after herself, she wasn't mentally able of cooking or cleaning and she needed constant prompting. There was no option of her returning home. (GP for Mrs Kent)

> I wasn't convinced that he'd manage back in the community, knowing what he's like - even with a home help or meals-on-wheels. (G.P. for Mr Mink)

3. *Residents felt inadequately or inappropriately supported*

Twenty one residents felt that the domiciliary care they received was not helpful in supporting them at home. A number of people thought the home help service providing one hour of home help per week, was too little and inappropriate to their needs, particularly for people in need of more personal support or constant attention. Some felt that such provision did little to overcome their fear of falling at night-time or their loneliness. One person suggested that a better solution would have been to employ a companion to live with him but no evidence was found of such an arrangement having been tried:

> What good is one hour of home help if you're lonely. (Mr Crille, The Orchard)

> I could have had a home help, but I didn't want someone else here where my wife had been doing things. Also I would still be left alone at night. (Mr Hockley, Elizabeth House)

The lack of support services for confused people was frequently mentioned as a reason why elderly people could not remain at home. This supports the finding in Chapter 5 that a number of confused people entered private care because of inadequate support networks:

> With her short term memory loss she would refuse meals, thinking she'd already eaten. I knew from a professional point of view there was a fear of exploitation and neighbours were very worried. Something had to be done. (Mrs Jones, The Dingle)

The lack of appropriate provision and support in order to stay at home was clearly evident in examples where there was an attempt at rehabilitation from hospital. Eighteen people, in settings other than their own home, (mainly hospitals) were not rehabilitated home because of lack of support. In several cases they experienced a trial period at home which broke down. The majority saw the brief trial period with an occupational therapist as unrealistic in assessing their ability to cope at home, and residents felt they were not and could not be given a chance to prove their ability, in a couple of hours or over a few days, particularly if they faced a change of circumstances, for example, the loss of carer through a bereavement at home:
I went home for one day to see if I could manage - I wouldn't have come here without doing that, but I couldn't cope. (Mrs Bacton, The Limes)

> The thought of a home help and being at home alone, I hated the most - I needed someone to talk to. (Miss Norwich, Millside)

> There was no alarm system, meals on wheels or home help over which we had control so I couldn't send her back as she kept wandering. (Social worker for Miss Corbin, Eaton Lodge)

Lack of confidence in their ability to return home was a major factor for a number of people that led to a breakdown in community care as an alternative option. Eighteen people gave this reason as to why they could not cope with going home. A choice between alternatives could also not be made unless the elderly person was aware of what options were available. Two people, for example, claimed they did not know of any community care provision to help them 'stay put':

The social worker didn't even mention community care. (Miss Johnson, The Rectory)

4. Residential care as a housing solution

Private residential care was used as an alternative housing option by some (14) who were homeless or were in a situation where their home was unsuitable to their needs or conditions, particularly if they were wheelchair-bound. Four of these people were already in other settings, for example, hospitals or other residential homes, and were unable to return to their former home. For others (2) their houses were in 'such a bad a state of repair' and beyond any 'acceptable' level of habitation.

> I can't really go home now I'm in a wheelchair. (Mrs Vickery, The Suffolk)

> The stairs meant I couldn't remain at home, whatever level of support. (Mr Bailey, The Lawns)

> I had no alternative as I had no other home to go back to. (Miss Short, The Risings)

> The social worker said I had no choice, I was homeless and needed the first vacancy. (Mr Kirk, The Dingle)

> She couldn't have stayed at home, it was like a death trap. (Social worker for Miss Sirus, The Suffolk). I agreed (resident).

In such conditions a move to residential care was a pragmatic response to circumstances faced, rather than a preference expressed by the elderly people themselves. One lady, however, chose private residential care as a housing option:

> I didn't want the upheaval of modernising my own home - I'd still be lonely. (Miss Prim, Inglenook)

Alternatives to enable Miss Prim to remain in the community may have been presented if this lady had sought admission via a professional. However, she found that alternative accommodation at the age of 89 meant waiting lists and contact with agencies holding different policies and criteria for different people. In this case, as in others, waiting lists operated as a perverse incentive to encourage admission into private residential care.

Community alternatives other than 'home'

1. Sheltered housing as an independent alternative. Overwhelmingly this option was not followed because elderly people and their relatives believed tenants in sheltered housing had to be fit and well and able to live independently, for example:

> This is a modern conception made for younger people in their 60's and 70's. Once you get to your 80's its not so good. (Miss Johnson, The Windmill)

> My daughter-in-law explored it as an option but I was too bad. (Mrs Crise, The Windmill)

A number of residents in one area expressed their wish to enter a particular private sheltered housing scheme which offered extra care facilities.

> The lack of finance and a long waiting list were barriers to this as a realistic alternative (Mrs Gould, Elizabeth House; Mr Gotts, Gracelands).

2. Living with relatives and friends in a domestic setting. Moving to live with family or friends was not considered by many as a realistic option. [Only 3 per cent (7) of residents stated that this was an option]. Although families generally supported elderly people in the community and were major contributors to their decision to enter a home, few elderly people expressed the desire or ability to share accommodation with their close relatives or 'burden them with extra care'. Relatives also disliked the idea for the following reasons.

There were competing interests among family members: some felt it was difficult to care for their parents and keep a full-time job; others were engaged in looking after other dependents (13).

> She really wanted to come and live with us but it was impossible, we have our own business. (Mrs Peters/The Limes, niece)

> She couldn't live with any other members of the family as we all have teenage children and they just don't mix - blaring music etc. When she went to live with another daughter for nine weeks, mother and son had to share a bedroom and the family situation became very fraught. (Daughter of Mrs Harris, The Rectory)

Other families were unable to care because of illness (9) or felt they could not cope, while a number of people faced difficult family relationships (6).

> She did come to live with us but it didn't work out as my wife found out she had Parkinson's disease. (Son of Mrs Hayman, Underwood)

Some of these residents felt bitter about the inability of their family to offer them an alternative:

> I still feel I oughtn't to have come, particularly with five children in their own homes - they just want their liberty after work. I never once thought my children wouldn't have me to live with them. (Mrs Keating, Limestone)

> She's been a nuisance ever since father died. She expects to come with us wherever we go. We don't go out much and our lives would lose

> spontaneity if she came to live with us. (Daughter)

Five families could not house their elderly relative because of accommodation difficulties. The lack of space in relatives' houses posed a problem for some:

> It would have been totally unsatisfactory as she would be sleeping on the settee. (Social worker for Mrs Muir, Seaview)

> We've only got one bedroom and we couldn't cope, particularly with her wandering at night. (Son of Mrs Joel, Hillside)

Three families were advised against accommodating their elderly relative by the G.P. or social worker.

Private v public residential care

Residential care was perceived as inevitable by the majority of elderly people in the study. However, Tables 6.1 and 6.2 showed that private sector residents (44 per cent v 34 per cent) had more choice of which residential home they entered than residents in the local authority sector, although this choice was constrained to the private sector alone.

A smaller number of these residents had the option of a local authority placement (8 per cent) or a variety of alternatives, consisting of a community care package, local authority residential care and another private home (10 per cent).

The choice for local authority residents was between a public and a private home. Few residents chose between a selection of public sector homes, choice within this system being inherently restricted through the bureaucratic process (see Literature Review).

Reasons for choosing private residential care

Table 6.6 shows that entry for the majority of residents to a private home was not through preference. A small number made a positive commitment to one particular sector but for the majority the move into private residential care was pragmatic because public sector places were seen to be restricted.

TABLE 6.6
REASONS FOR DECIDING BETWEEN PUBLIC AND PRIVATE RESIDENTIAL CARE

	No.	%
Local authority home an option		
1. Rejected consciously	21	10
2. Influenced by relatives/professionals against Local authority home	6	3
3. Distance deterred entry	2	1
4. No reason specified	6	3
	35	17
Local authority home not an option		
Unable to pursue because:		
Lack of vacancy etc.	76	38
distance	15	7
professional decided against it	20	10
not aware of local authority home	10	5
would not have chosen even if it were an option	20	10
No reason given	24	13
	165	83

Thirty-five people (17 per cent) in the private sector thought they could have gained admission to local authority accommodation. Of these, 21 consciously decided between public and private residential care. A minority of residents, therefore, opted in favour of private care and did not entertain any consideration of a local authority home. The main reason for this hinged upon the elderly persons or their relatives' perception of local authority homes as not providing what they really wanted (Diagram 6.1).

DIAGRAM 6.1
RESIDENTS' CHOICE OF PUBLIC OR PRIVATE RESIDENTIAL CARE

> I didn't want a public home, I only wanted private. (Mrs Brookman, Conifers)

> A Local Authority residential home was unspeakable, I'd never consider or think about it - I'd already made the decision. (Mrs Elliot, The Yarmouth)

> I've had the experience of three council homes, it's OK but there aren't any carpets and as they (public and private) are the same price, I'd rather be a private patient. I'm not used to their class of people. (Miss Saunders, Seaview)

> I don't want mother sitting around the walls or sharing a bedroom. (Daughter of Mrs Goodyear, Hillside)

> I moved around quite a lot and went several times to a Local Authority residential home. Anyway I hated it - residents there just weren't with it and I had to pay for it too. (Miss Comet, The Rectory)

> My son-in-law had worked in one on a voluntary basis and didn't like it - he said they were a load of geriatrics. (Mr Dodson, aged 90, The Windmill)

> My sister-in-laws father went there and it wasn't clean. (Mrs Keating, Limestone)

The lack of privacy and stimulation thought to be present in local authority residential homes were two important features frequently voiced by relatives and residents alike, for not pursuing a public sector alternative:

> I spent a whole day in a local authority residential home. It just wasn't exciting - people sitting in chairs with their mouths hanging open. (Mrs Hurn, Rosehill)

The variety and mixture of different kinds of residents was not the only important consideration in rejecting public sector residential care. Some saw the local authority only catering for the 'down and outs' or confused and did not see themselves fitting in alongside. The inability to take personal items of furniture or a dog, ruled out public care as an option for some people. Some had other unpleasant memories:

> A local authority residential home had to be ruled out as father died in one in 1971. Mother has always been emotionally distressed by her mental picture of the place even now. (Daughter of Mrs Shotter, Underwood)

Reversing a number of these comments shows that people looking for a residential home sought elements of stimulation, company, some room to themselves and somewhere 'nice and comfortable' - all of which they felt could not be found in a local authority home.

Eight people also rejected public care because they were financially better off in a private home and a further three people rejected public care outright on political grounds or because they felt they would not fit in with 'that class of people'. All three were able-bodied people with the ability to choose between a variety of private homes.

These comments illustrate the minority of people who consciously rejected public sector residential care. However, a further 20 people for whom public sector care was not an option, said they would have rejected it if it had been available to them and gave similar reasons as those above.

For 83 per cent of the sample, public sector accommodation and care was not an option that could be followed (Table 6.6). Thirty eight percent of residents entered private residential care because they felt excluded from local authority residential homes through the lack of vacancies.

The move to private care was therefore pragmatic because public sector places were seen to be restricted and 'waiting lists' were perceived to be too long.

Thirty people said they would have accepted a placement in the local authority sector if a vacancy had existed at the time. Some or most of such vacancies pursued, however, were in particular homes, which were often very popular:

> We wanted her to go to Parklands, as I could easily slip in and visit her there, but there were no vacancies. This was the only other one nearby. (Daughter of Mrs Glamorgan, The Bridge)

In some cases, an admission to public sector care could not be arranged quickly enough.

> In the private home we had more freedom about when we entered. (Mr and Mrs Bakewell, The Suffolk)

The distance of the home from the local town acted as a barrier also for fifteen people. This particularly affected those people who suffered from advanced senile dementia and who had to move to out of town locations because of the lack of suitable provision in the vicinity.

> I knew she would have had to go out of the district - our EMI block here couldn't cope with confused wanderers. (Social worker for Miss Corbin, Eaton Lodge)

The evidence suggests, therefore, that the choice of a local authority residential home was blocked off mainly because of the public sector's inflexibility to respond to elderly people's needs and requests to enter residential care at a time and place suitable to them, or to match their expectations of residential care.

In other cases, it was a professional acting as 'gatekeeper' to public sector resources who restricted access to this sector because they felt the elderly person was not suitable or eligible for residential care. The only way Mrs Limp (The Bridge) from Surrey could live near her son was to look at a selection of private homes. In two other instances, County policy of not accepting financial responsibility for out-of-county residents excluded a local authority placement.

Not only were CPNs and social workers excluding residents from local authority residential homes for a variety of professional reasons but some, with a personal preference for private care, excluded access to other public resources such as home helps and directed people to the private sector (see Chapter 8).

> I went ahead with the local authority residential home but as she owned her own house and could clearly afford it, I thought she should go into private care. (Social Worker for Miss Elliston, Fenlands)

Another small group of people (10) never thought about public care because they were unaware they were eligible. All ten felt they were unfit for a council home.

> There was no mention of a council home. My health is no good and I could only go out in a chair ... I guess that's why I couldn't go. (Mrs Carlton, The Suffolk)

A further twenty four gave no reason for pursuing a course towards private residential care.

Local authority residents: public v private care

Local authority residents had little choice within the public sector. Only 23 per cent of local authority residents had the option of entering another local authority residential home (Table 6.1). There was nothing unusual about this group of people.

Why was there restricted choice in the public sector? This has already been covered in relation to private sector residents, but a glimpse at the qualitative evidence given by public sector residents shows very similar reasons why they too did not have a choice of local authority residential homes.

The public sector was never initially designed and was never intended to give elderly people a choice of home and as a result individual preferences in the decision-making, allocation and rationing processes count for little. With the pressure on local authority resources, also, when and where elderly people entered care depended on the vacancy state. Ten people found that when it came to a decision about entering a home there were no vacancies in any other local authority residential homes:

> I was going to Parklands but it was full up. They offered me this alternative. I was disappointed as I liked it there ... I'm used to this now. (Mrs Delves, Condor House)

> The local authority residential home I wanted was chock a block - the EMI unit there would have been ideal but it was Hobson's choice. (Social worker for Mr Carter, Wilmonton)

Entry to a particular local authority residential home may, therefore, be more through chance and less through the choice and the preference of the elderly person and their offspring. Some people were unable to enter the environment with which they had become familiar through regular short-term stays or day care, because of the lack of a permanent bed.

> She went to Richey House for short-term care, but they have very few permanent vacancies. You can state a preference, but there's nothing you can do if they are full up. (Sister of Miss Drew, The Grange)

The local authority sector was too inflexible to respond to their need at the right time and in the preferred place. Preferences formed a very small part of the allocation system and were not reflected in the eventual outcome of many residents. Only thirteen people (11 per cent) were able to enter their first choice of home.

Although residents were assessed as being in need of residential care, they were not guaranteed an appropriate setting to match their need because of the lack of suitable vacancies.

For potential residents who stated a preference for a particular home and stuck to their request, the wait for a vacancy was long.

> They've recently offered me a place at Wilmonton (six months after application) but I'm settled here now and don't see why I should move. (Mrs Jewson, Richey House)

People were also unable to choose local authority homes outside geographically determined boundaries. The pressure on beds was increased because of the factor of locality, a constraint not applicable in the private sector. In two other instances, the professional social worker advised against the nearest home and sought a placement elsewhere in the County.

There was also evidence of officers-in-charge operating restrictive practices and refusing to have residents returning from hospital. Some local authority residential homes refused re-admission after a hospital stay for 12 people. Most of these were confused and were often channelled into a specialist EMI unit.

> She was so confused she worried all the other residents. The ordinary local authority residential home couldn't cope. She was admitted to hospital for her own safety, but to stay there was unnecessary as she was untreatable. Although inappropriate to move her she had to go. She was under a guardianship order ... We could have looked at private EMI but we couldn't set it up quick enough. (Social worker for Miss Pinker, The Lodge)

There was also evidence to suggest people returning from hospital in wheelchairs were being placed in alternative homes:

My room was upstairs and so I couldn't return in a wheelchair. (Mr Burnham/Sideview)

Why did most public sector residents not have the option of private care? The majority of local authority residents (77 per cent) felt excluded from the private sector. Thirty three (27 per cent) felt this because they believed that admission to the private sector would have been financially impossible.

We had to lower our expectations when we realised the financial position. (Social worker for Miss Davies, Sheringham)

Meanwhile they wanted a £600 deposit. I immediately advised against it. (Social worker for Mrs Almey, Parklands)

Although he owned the house, his money wouldn't see him through private care. (Social worker for Mr Bunting, The Cliffs)

In two cases the family deterred their elderly parent from looking to the private sector because they feared they would be made financially responsible. A further fourteen people (12 per cent) were excluded as vacancies were not available at the time of crisis and the available accommodation was not suitable for 8 further people (7 per cent):

I couldn't find one that would take them both as each had different needs - he needed nursing care and she was in a wheelchair. (Social worker for Mr and Mrs Pope, Sheringham)

Nine people were rejected because of their age, physical condition or their mental state and for four others distance deterred entry. Another group of people (13) rejected private care out of preference, some being politically against the privatisation of care and 'exploitation of elderly people for profit'.

In five instances it was the relatives who expressed a prejudice against private care.

We disregarded private care because we expected it to be awful. (Relative of Miss Crimp, The Cliffs)

In seven cases social workers also exercised professional judgements over the suitability of placing elderly people in particular private homes:

She comes from a family well known to social services and we know no private home would welcome her family trooping through. (Social worker for Mrs Cane, The Lodgings)

I didn't feel we could place her in any of the private homes here as no one could cope with her level of dementia. We did look at one in particular but we would have infringed their registration as there were too many demented people there anyway. (Social worker for Mrs Jarvis, The Grange)

Finally, thirteen other residents (11 per cent) said that they just did not consider private care, because they did not know of its existence.

In contrast to those who felt excluded from private care, twenty nine local authority residents said that they had the option of living in a private sector home. So why did they not pursue it? Thirteen residents expressed a preference for the home or sector they were in, one relative influenced the decision of another resident; for three people the vacancy did not materialise; for another six finances made the eventual move to a private home impossible. Finally, a further six were rejected after a trial stay in a private home because of their age or mental condition.

Alternative choice within the private sector

Seventy two elderly people in the private sector (36 per cent) had a choice of two or more private homes. Why did they reject or not enter some homes?

A number of people were excluded by factors such as high fees (1) or were rejected by the home owner (5):

> No other homes would take him. He was rejected by many because they knew him to be a homosexual. He was incontinent and terminally ill so very dependent. Others didn't want to know. (Mr Stewart, The Dingle, home owner)

Three other homes failed to accommodate three residents because they were unable to manage their mental state. Such residents had already been rejected or refused readmission from other private homes. Homeless, the relative sought the first available vacancy in a specialist home for the elderly mentally infirm.

Some residents made a conscious decision to reject certain private homes because of their isolated location (10) or because they could not provide a vacancy at the appropriate time (20).

> We looked at two other homes at the point of her departure from hospital ... but there were no vacancies at either. (Nephew of Mr Gringle, The Bridges)

Thirty three people (45 per cent of those who had the option of another private home) rejected the alternative home because either they or their relatives did not like the home or its staff. Several reasons were given:

1. In some homes the accommodation was unsuitable as it meant sharing or the layout did not suit their circumstances, particularly if they were in a wheelchair.

> We made lots of enquiries but we had great difficulty in finding one suitable as most had no downstairs accommodation for wheelchairs. In fact we tried all the homes in a 10-15 mile radius over two months. They often said yes, but we'd go back and still be bottom of the list as the vacancy wasn't on the ground floor. I went back to one home ten times

and they had no vacancies ... I also got the feeling they'd all prefer women. (Sister-in-law of Mr Price, The Rest)

2. One of the main areas of dissatisfaction voiced by residents concerned the assortment of residents. This feature of a home could only be experienced on admission and was difficult to anticipate prior to entry.

Many of the negative comments centred around the experience of loneliness within the private home, particularly in situations where they were expected to 'integrate' with other residents, especially those who were confused and with whom they could not hold a conversation.

For some, mixing with others was a completely new and threatening experience, particularly as many were living alone prior to admission.

> Living with other people is difficult - you can't join in if you don't know how to. (Mrs Payne, The Copse)

The lack of stimulation was another feature of unhappiness. Eight per cent of people interviewed confirmed a finding in the research undertaken by Willcocks et al (1985) that the residential environment exerted 'too few demands on the elderly person leading to maladaptive behaviour, such as boredom and apathy'.

3. Relatives vetoed a number of options on behalf of the elderly person, for example:

> I didn't take to the home as soon as I saw it, so I ruled it out. (Niece of Mrs Peters, The Limes)

4. In some homes, there was a particular stigma attached:

> No one speaks well of it, there's no freedom and I wouldn't choose it. (Mrs Howlett, Gracelands)

Although residential care was inevitable there were some, therefore, who were able to exercise a choice - mainly those able to entertain the private sector as an option where there was real choice between a range of homes and it was here that preferences could be expressed.

The market attraction of private homes

The home owners' existence depended on their ability to convince relatives and their parents that they could offer an acceptable quality of life, not only in relation to other homes, but in contrast to the local authority sector. So far this chapter has shown that people were not making choices between different sectors of care, but between competing private homes.

All participants in the study were asked what made them choose that particular private or local authority home. Table 6.7 records the primary reason given for their selection.

TABLE 6.7
WHY THIS PARTICULAR HOME?

	Private		Local Authority	
	No.	%	No.	%
Reason				
Vacancy	44	22	46	38
Other person (mainly relatives) liked the home	42	21	2	2
Elderly person liked the home	28	14	16	13
Recommended	22	11	-	-
Home located near to friends/ relatives	22	11	22	18
Elderly person previously lived nearby	14	7	22	18
Other	20	10	4	3
Not known	8	4	8	7
	200	100	120	100

Table 6.7 shows that relatives were able to exercise their preferences between homes in the private sector of care to a great extent. Relatives were, therefore, empowered not only to take decisions but to select particular homes. Only 14 per cent of residents exercised positive choice in the selection of a home.

What were potential residents and their relatives seeking in a private home? Both residents and their relatives selected homes on the basis of similar features such as location, size and atmosphere.

Locational factors were very important in their selection; especially important was the general attractiveness of the area in which the home was situated. To some the location was attractive because they had already lived in the area for several years and had built up a network of friends and relatives with whom they could maintain contact. Others returned to an area they had visited on holiday. The situational features of the home, whether it overlooked the sea, had gardens, or was near the church or shops, were influential considerations in decision-making.

These marketable factors were also influential in the home owners' reasons for purchasing.

I saw it in the yellow pages. By the address I knew it was near the sea

> and the hospital as I used to come here for holidays. (Mrs Gowling, Gracelands)

Particularly important for local inhabitants, were the reputations of homes, owners and their staff which spread via word of mouth in the area. On this basis very few home owners advertised nationally. Although few chose homes primarily and solely on recommendation, this factor played a significantly greater part in the selection of private homes than in the selection of homes in the Local Authority sector.

The home itself in terms of atmosphere and size were paramount factors in the residents' and relatives' judgement of a suitable home. Residents looked for a friendly and homely atmosphere, which they often found in the smaller sized homes.

For residential homes to be competitive they also needed to offer privacy in the form of single rooms. This was yet another attractive feature of private homes, seducing potential residents to this sector of care. Nearly all the 39 homes offered single accommodation and some advertised extra en suite facilities: the availability of a private bathroom, however, captured only those who could pay extra.

Some residents and relatives only selected private homes where there was a degree of flexibility to accommodate individual personal needs, for example by allowing dogs to remain on the premises, permitted smoking in rooms or provided special facilities for wheelchair users. Individual room space catered for individual tastes to some extent - and was an important consideration in the residents' judgement of a particular home. Breakfast in bed was mentioned by one man in his selection of a home!

Finally security, particularly during the night, was a major consideration and was important to the relatives. Many elderly people themselves however were relieved by the knowledge that someone else was on hand if they needed help.

> There is night attention. They bring me a cup of tea and take me to the toilet. That's why I chose it in the first place. (Mrs Vickery, The Suffolk)

Twenty two per cent of residents had the opportunity to enter a particular home simply because a vacancy existed. They did not primarily select it on attractiveness but because it could accommodate them at the right point in time. In such cases, it was often the relative who selected the home rather than the elderly person.

> The hospital phoned to say they had found a vacancy - we went straight away to see the place and liked it so said yes there and then. (Relative of Mrs Glamorgan, The Bridges)

On reflection the majority of residents and their relatives were happy with the 'package' of residential care chosen.

This study did not attempt to look at 'outcome' in terms of the level of adjustment to residential care (for further details see Booth, 1985; Davies and Knapp, 1981), but it did capture a consumer viewpoint from the residents interviewed in relation to their new physical and social environment.

Resident satisfaction

Subjective measures and general questions related to residents' satisfaction is beset with problems both in explanation and interpretation: some of these have been highlighted in Chapter Two.

Despite the difficulties two main checks were employed in the questionnaire to check consistency of response - one included the interviewer's assessment of mood on a 5 point scale; the other directly asked the resident how they felt about the future. Only the levels of satisfaction and happiness are considered in this chapter.

Table 6.8 records the response of residents to the question 'Are you satisfied with services in this home?'

TABLE 6.8
RESIDENTS' SATISFACTION WITH SERVICES IN PRIVATE HOMES

	No.	%
Very satisfied	50	25
Satisfied	80	40
Neutral	30	15
Not satisfied	10	5
Not known (i.e. confused/answer refused)	30	15
	200	100

This measure of well being was followed by a question rating happiness with life in general. Table 6.9 records response to the question 'Are you happy with your life at present?'

TABLE 6.9
RESIDENTS' HAPPINESS WITH LIFE IN PRIVATE HOMES

	No.	%
Very happy	20	10
Happy	80	40
Neutral	56	28
Unhappy	14	7
Not known	30	15
	200	100

These figures show that the majority of elderly people were satisfied with the services on offer in the private home in which they were resident and were happy with their life at the point of interview. The interviewer's assessment of mood confirmed this finding.

On closer examination, residents indicated four areas which related to their measures of satisfaction and happiness; these could be grouped into elements of staff care, which reflected positive responses and elements of 'resident mix' and adjustment to residential life reflecting negative features (Table 6.10). The latter captured a view of how well the resident felt they had adjusted to their new environment.

TABLE 6.10
FACTORS ASSOCIATED WITH HAPPINESS AND SATISFACTION

Main factors identified	Positive Response %	Negative Response %
Caring	10	5
Services	20	2
Resident mix	6	9
Life in general: 'adjustment to residential life'	10	23
Unknown	15	
	46	39

Satisfaction with the caring aspects of home life included statements related to the kindness and industriousness of staff, particularly where they were on call twenty four hours of the day. Good food and hotel type service were other major parts of the package on which consumers based their assessment along with the charm and comfort of the physical environment. Similar factors were considered in the professional's view of the 39 private homes (Diagram 6.2).

DIAGRAM 6.2
PROFESSIONAL VIEWS OF PRIVATE HOMES STUDIED

Negative comments:

1. ENVIRONMENTAL:
   - Would be better if they had single rooms
   - The architecture is very difficult - it's not suitable
   - Badly situated for the shops - dead

2. SERVICES:
   - Not enough staff to give individual attention

3. CARING:
   - They have a quick turnover - will take anyone and try and cope

4. ATMOSPHERE:
   - Too many confused there. Not the place if you're OK.

Positive comments:

1. ENVIRONMENTAL:
   - Attractive with separate dining room
   - Always immaculate
   - It's purpose built

2. SERVICES:
   - Well furnished and the food is good

3. CARING:
   - Excellent, will take people with problems and cope
   - You only have to step inside to see how caring they are
   - Real personal care
   - The matron coped more than adequately. Her judgement and treatment of the behaviour of the client were such that the client settled and was happy.

4. ATMOSPHERE:
   - It's homely, better than a local authority residential home.

Residents scores were amalgamated to form an overall score per home. Three groups of homes were found:

1. In 64 per cent (25) of homes, <u>all</u> the residents were happy with life and satisfied with the 'package' offered;

2. In 28 per cent (11) there were a majority of happy and satisfied residents;

3. Only in 8 per cent (3) of homes were the majority of residents unhappy and dissatisfied.

Other alternatives

1. Unregistered private homes were considered by four.

2. Nursing homes were investigated by another four people who eventually came into private residential care. The dividing line between a nursing care home and residential care home confused residents, and some rejected or were rejected by nursing homes because they found the environment of illness depressing and frightening or they were too fit.

3. Alternative hospital provision was also not possible for a number on the grounds that they were not in need of constant medical care and attention or where long term psychiatric hospitals were concerned, the policy of community care greatly reduced the number of beds available.

The market model of welfare allows for positive choice

This section examines the proposition that the effective choice of services by consumers of welfare was greater in the private sector than in the public sector.

In theory, the great advantage of the market system is that it enhances individual freedom to exercise personal preference and allows for self-determination, free from professional and bureaucratic hurdles faced by the public sector (Chapter One). In practice this means that elderly people could select between a variety of residential homes in the private sector to a greater extent than they could in the public sector.

Unlike the private sector, the public sector was not designed to take into account individual preferences. As a result the flexibility to exercise preference and move within the system was constrained by the allocation system which offered provision on a 'take it' or 'leave it' basis.

The notion of choice was a central marketing feature of the private sector and with the boom in private residential homes it was presumed that a greater number of people would be able to exercise that choice. The argument that residents have more choice in their future direction of care via the market model was also a justification for the increase in state support to those financially unable but wanting to enter private care.

The concept of choice, defined as the opportunity of choosing from alternative actions or possibilities, is, however, too simplistic a notion in relation to elderly people entering residential care in both free market and welfare models. There were a number of constraints in exercising a realistic and effective choice, regardless of the eventual sector offering care. The expression of choice was not free in either sector - home owners in the private sector had the right of veto over every admission while the bureaucratic process deflected choice in the public sector. The ability to pay allowed the private sector resident choice between homes, irrespective of need, in a way which would not have been possible for those without adequate funds.

Chapter Four also illustrated that not all residents were able to exercise choice in entering a private home because they were confused and incapable of deciding for themselves. Physical frailty also excluded a small number of people from exercising free market choice, because certain homes deterred wheelchair users, through their layout or because of their admission policy.

Selecting between various possibilities required time as well as ability. Although the majority planned their admission, only a few had time available to carefully proceed through the transition from home into residential care. If a crisis arose or pressure was exerted on those people in scarce hospital beds, relatives very often took the first appropriate vacancy they could find.

Information about alternatives was also far from perfect. Some did not consider or investigate alternatives because of the negative perceptions and expectations they held about certain provision. Advertising of provision was scarce, and in some cases (particularly the public sector) non-existent: in addition few people engaged a specialist to discuss the pros and cons of such options.

Relatives collected a range of information on private homes but the real test of a home could only be undertaken by the resident. However, once in the home, the opportunity to select another home was not easy, so the supermarket model could not be directly applied to residential care. This study also confirmed that there was little movement between homes once residents were admitted. Although theoretically, therefore, there was an element of choice in the private sector, choice was not simply given to people by increasing the provision of private care.

Bearing in mind the various constraints on resident choice in both sectors, the evidence presented in this chapter supports the argument that choice was greater in the private sector. By drawing on this evidence, the various stages in the process of admission are examined in light of the alternatives open to potential residents of both sectors.

For the majority in both sectors the stark choice between remaining at home or entering a residential setting did not exist - residential care was unavoidable. For those in the local authority sector not only were there few community options but virtually no choice between residential settings. For those in the private sector community options were similarly restricted but there was apparent choice between different private homes.

A small number of private sector residents opted for residential care out of preference but the majority entered because community care resources were either unavailable - even for those with financial means - or unacceptable and did not suit their needs. In light of the emphasis placed on community care in terms of planning and policy making, this finding is of significance.

In relation to choice between public and private care, again few people exercised a preference but entered for pragmatic reasons. People entered the sector of care where they thought there were vacancies. However, customers of private sector provision did have some choice in the private home they entered. Local authority residents were much more constrained in exercising the same degree of choice through the lack of vacancies in their sector.

From the series of interviews we can see what attracted elderly people and (more significantly for the home owners) their relatives to particular private homes. Attractive surroundings and a familiar neighbourhood were important external features; a good reputation helped, along with an emphasis on security. Such were the features which were important to relatives. In addition, privacy, atmosphere and a flexible regime to cater for individual tastes were paramount in the decisions of both relative and resident.

The person exercising such choice in the private sector, however, may not always be the elderly person, but as this study shows (Chapter Eight) was more likely to be a relative. The customer, therefore, may not be the direct consumer. Evidence showed that it was often a third party who was influential in the decision-making and it was often the preferences of these indirect consumers that were expressed. Such a scenario was particularly true for those elderly people coming from hospital.

The evidence from this chapter shows that residential care was inevitable, but with the involvement of relatives a variety of private homes could be explored.

Whether elderly people themselves chose or whether the decision to enter was taken by another person, whether there existed a preference to enter private residential care or whether it was a variety of circumstances that determined entry, the majority of people were happy and satisfied with their eventual outcome.

The growth of private residential care has given people choice over location, size and standards. The variety of provision within this sector, illustrated in Chapter Three provided some real alternatives in the kind of provision available and did not just present different packaging to the same provision. For example, residential care was not only found in a small domestic home or a large purpose built home but there were differences in 'regime' and style of management as well as philosophy of care which provided different kinds of care. A genuine choice therefore existed.

In practice, however, only the minority of residents were able to take advantage of this situation and exercise genuine choice.

Admission to private and public homes appeared not to be through choice and preference. Only 21 (11 per cent) private residential care residents consciously opted for the private sector and 13 (11 per cent) local authority residents opted for the public sector.

Together this illustrates that only 11 per cent (34) of elderly people made a commitment to one sector or the other. For 89 per cent of elderly people the choice was restricted.

Two similar systems of residential care exist side by side with very similar populations entering via similar routes. The final decision to enter private or public residential care, was pragmatic rather than an expression of preference.

The assessment of genuine choice between and within the sectors is problematic and complex. Such difficulty led the Wagner Committee to report that:

> Choice is no longer the simple process of a potential resident choosing from alternative services, it becomes a process of negotiation of which the key feature has to be honesty in analysing the comparative needs of the parties involved ... In the end, one or more of the parties may be a loser in the sense that the outcome may not coincide with their personal choice, but the process, if successful, will lead to a positive consensus. (Wagner, 1988, p.9)

Negotiation between all parties involved in the admission leading to a positive consensus may be a more realistic definition of choice in the process of admission. The next chapter looks at the process of negotiation between key operators in the admission and discusses further the notion of consumer choice.

7 Key operators in the process of admission: home owners and their selection process

The expansion of private sector provision over the last decade was advocated in terms of extending personal freedom and increasing individual responsibility while enhancing consumer choice (Chapter One). On the basis of these three claims, the Thatcher government poured in vast amounts of public money to make available such alternative provision. Choice between public and private residential sectors was and still is seen as a marketable quality (Chapter Six).

However, certain suppositions govern choice - one of which is that choice lies in the hands of the purchaser, in this case, the elderly person who enters private residential care. Principles of the market, however, can be applied less readily to the arena of residential care than to a customer in a shop. Chapters Five and Six illustrated that admission was seldom a carefully thought out process with a choice between a number of possible and available alternatives - it was often due to an accumulation of circumstances with the consumer having very little control over events. Chapters Seven and Eight reveal that other people are significant in the process of admission. The relationship between key operators often suggests that elderly people are the least powerful to exercise choice in the area of their future care.

The ultimate choice lies in the hands of one person - the home owner who could admit or reject a particular person on the basis of their decision alone.

This Chapter looks at the home owners' assessment and selection process and discusses the factors important in their decision-making.

Thirty-nine homes were visited and, in each case, a home owner or manager was interviewed regarding their role in the process. They were asked to describe the necessary requirements in order to gain entry into their home and to outline the various stages in the admission process. Two main conclusions can be stated on the basis of the evidence.

1. At the time of the research the home owner made the key decision on whether or not to admit an elderly person to their home. Although home owners depended on the market system to make their business viable, there was evidence that demand exceeded supply. Consequently home owners could select residents and choose to admit or reject anyone: in other words, they held the power of veto over any resident.

The home owner could also ignore professional opinion; for they were neither totally dependent upon social workers nor general practitioners for their referrals or their financial support. Although relatives were significant influences, even their views were treated with caution.

With changes in the economy and market pressures the situation is likely to change, with home owners having less choice in who they accept or reject as they attempt to keep their businesses viable by filling all vacant beds. Changes with the Community Care Act 1990 will also mean a professional assessment for those requiring Income Support, giving professional social workers more say in the admission of a major group of residents.

2. The factors considered in a home owner's assessment were different from those used by professional social workers operating in the process - a person's ability to pay and their medical history were of paramount importance in the eyes of most home owners.

The role of the home owner in the process of admission

The selection process of residents in studies of local authority residential allocation was found to be as important as the characteristics of the elderly people themselves in determining who was allocated a residential home place (Paterson, 1978; Ovenstone and Bean, 1981). This section looks at the various stages in the selection process as seen by the thirty-nine home owners. It is interesting to note three common features throughout the stages of admission:

1. Home owners took on two major roles in the selection process - as gatekeepers and assessors.

2. The purpose of the home owner's assessment and the factors they used in assessing prospective residents were different from those operated by the social workers in the study.

3. The relationship between home owners and professionals in the field was also varied and complex. Some home owners chose to ignore the views of significant professionals and took it upon themselves to assess for suitability without professional guidance (see Chapter Eight).

The stages of admission

Diagram 7.1 illustrates the stages of admission as seen from the home owner's perspective. At least four of the five stages were outlined by 90 per cent of owners, each marking a step further in the process to becoming a 'successful' applicant. At each step the home owner had the option to pass the potential resident on to the next stage.

Stage 1. The referral - home owner as advertiser and promoter of private provision. Thirty one of the 39 owners felt the crucial factor in sales promotion was the reputation of the home, which was generally spread by word of mouth among local people and professionals. Local networks and personal contacts were felt to be more effective for publicity than large-scale advertising campaigns (13 homes advertised nationally but the majority of people who entered private residential care were from a local catchment area). 'Getting it right at the initial contact' was therefore crucial in the promotion of business.

The importance of a good local reputation was reflected in the source of referral. Home owners were asked about their major sources of referrals and Table 7.1 illustrates these.

TABLE 7.1
SOURCE OF REFERRALS

	No.	%
Relative	31	79
Social worker	29	74
GP	22	56
Resident (self)	5	13
Solicitor	2	5
Friend	2	5

(number of home owners = 39)

DIAGRAM 7.1
STAGES OF ADMISSION INTO PRIVATE RESIDENTIAL CARE: HOME OWNERS' PERSPECTIVE

Unsuccessful applicant		Successful applicant
Stage 1 May be given a list of other homes and vacancies and/or placed on waiting list	PHONE REFERRAL	1. Exchange of information between home owner and referrer 2. Resident assessed with regard to physical state and financial means 3. Brochure sent
Stage 2 Relative may decide home not suitable	RELATIVE VISITS	Sharing information
Stage 3 Resident rejects home	RESIDENT VISITS OR IS VISITED	1. Chance for resident to see the home 2. Assessment by home owner 3. Care requirements discussed Home owner may consult 'others' 'assessments'
Stage 4 Resident rejects home	TRIAL PERIOD	1. Test out/check difficulties 2. Opportunity for resident to settle and 'forget about the past'
Stage 5 Resident rejects homes	CONTRACT	1. Agreement between home owner and resident to mark 'permanent' resident 2. Rules and regulations for resident 3. Indication of services on offer 4. Protection for resident and home owner

The initial referral generally came via a telephone call, mainly from a relative enquiring about the availability of residential provision or from a professional who may have already assessed the person for purposes of a public sector placement. (With the reduction in local authority places as local authorities sell off their residential provision, the referral rate to the private sector could increase.)

The role of the home owner at this point of referral was crucial - they had no role to play if there were no vacancies in their home although some owners redirected people to other homes or placed people on a waiting list for the next available room. Alternatively, if there was a vacancy they promoted and advertised their provision at this point of contact.

There was little evidence of home owners touting for business (one home - The Suffolk) with only two homes routinely contacting social workers or other professionals when a vacancy arose; these were homes which admitted very confused residents.

An exchange of information between the home owner and referring agent took place at this stage also. Thirteen home owners thought that their main function was to share details of the home with relatives or professionals and explore the reasons for admission. The initial referral stage was the main assessment stage for five homes (13 per cent): at The Lawns, the owner stated 'we assess immediately for fitness'.

Stage 2. Home owner as host. In seven homes, the next formal stage consisted of an invitation for the *relatives only* to visit in order to exchange detailed information 'with as little inconvenience to the potential resident as possible'.

Stage 3. Home owner as assessor. At each stage the majority of home owners assessed the suitability of the prospective resident in terms of whether she and her staff could cope with the level of disability or presenting problem.

The initial assessment in Stage 1 was primarily a time to gather such details and assess the elderly person's physical and mental state as well as to discuss the financial arrangements concerned with the placement. These factors in assessment are discussed later in this chapter.

In the sequence of events, the visit of the potential customer or resident to the home formed the main 'formal' assessment period, particularly in terms of sociability, resident mix, behavioral and other social factors. Twenty six home owners (66 per cent) required the prospective resident either to visit the home and, if possible, to stay for one day; or the home owners themselves visited the prospective resident in their home environment or in hospital.

This stage provided a forum for exchange of information, yet twenty home owners (51 per cent) saw this time mainly for their own purposes to continue assessment (this was often not made clear to the resident) and to discuss the care requirements of the resident:

> We talk informally and I'm assessing all the time. (Brookside)
>
> We'll have a look at them, tell them about the routine and ask questions of their medical history which makes up our assessment. (The Yarmouth)

Some home owners felt their assessment to be sufficient, while others, before making a decision to accept or reject a prospective resident, went a step further and consulted 'outside' opinion and called for a formal assessment by the person's general practitioner or social worker. This appeared to depend on whether an 'outside' agency was already involved with the prospective resident or had established links with the home, and whether the home owner saw this as a necessary step in helping them come to a decision. Without these three factors, it was less likely that a second opinion was called for. Only nine home owners (23 per cent) required a reference from another source as a necessary requirement in their process of admission.

Stage 4. Home owner as decision-maker. Thirty five home owners (90 per cent) accepted or rejected the client formally after their assessment. The objective of the following stage of a trial period was to assess the difficulties encountered by the resident within the home. However, four homes (10 per cent) accepted the potential resident on a trial basis immediately following Stage 1.

The final decision was taken during a trial period which, in twenty five homes (64 per cent), lasted one month, although this varied in the other fourteen homes from two weeks to six months. Residents likely to be rejected at this stage were those who displayed violent and aggressive behaviour, particularly if it affected other residents; those residents with management problems, or those people not accepted by other residents, in one example, a recent stroke victim.

Although some home owners said that once they had accepted a resident they kept him or her for as long as possible, twenty six owners recollected occasions of rejecting residents. The onset of senile dementia (often with accompanying aggressive and physically abusive behaviour) to the extent that staff were unable to cope was the most frequent reason for rejection after admission. Other applicants likely to be rejected included those who suffered a psychotic illness or were defined as being in need of 'nursing home' care. This suggests that the home owners' assessments were not always correct or complete. Medical factors were important from the outset but sociability was difficult to judge at the initial stages unless a trial period or short-term stay was arranged. Those residents who were rejected due to anti-social behaviour were almost always rejected after admission.

Although a variety of provision was on offer for different kinds of elderly people, confused or not, the majority of home owners were homogeneous in the kind of client they rejected.

Stage 5. Home owner as contractor of care. The final role in the process came after admission when the terms of agreement or contract was signed symbolizing the elderly person's status as a permanent resident. Eleven home owners (28 per cent) marked this passage through the admission process by the signing of a contract and a further eleven by giving terms and conditions of residence to all residents and relatives.

Factors in assessment

Assessment for admission into public sector residential care involved a multi-faceted approach as a basis for decision-making and planning a mode of life after admission. In such an assessment in the public sector a range of factors were considered based on the *need* for residential care. Such provision was for:

> Elderly people, who after careful assessment of their medical and social needs, were unable to maintain themselves in their own homes, even with the support from outside...and not in need of continuous care by nursing staff. (DHSS, 1972, p.12)

This assessment involved other agencies as well as social services, in collecting information on clients' circumstances, their financial, medical, social and personal history, their network of relationships and presenting problems. The prospective resident may view such public sector assessment as another step in the invasion of their privacy and turn to the private sector because it does not necessarily call for such 'in-depth' intrusion. The Suffolk study, however, found that home owners employed their own form of assessment, the three main factors in selection of residents concerning the financial, physical and social well-being of residents.

Financial factors

This section does not attempt to look at the value for money related to quality or quantity of service but looks at the financial factors considered in the assessment process. The whole of the private sector is distinguished by its cash nexus - the exchange of welfare services for a payment - and is governed by the individual's ability to pay for the service he or she receives.

Unlike entry to public sector residential care, there was no requirement in the private sector for a professional assessment of need because market forces operated to ration and allocate resources based on the ability to pay.

Eligibility in a free market rested on financial considerations and even those seeking state support through the supplementary benefit system were not required to demonstrate their need for such provision as long as they had below £3,000 in capital assets (based on 1986 figures) and insufficient income. Again, in contrast to public sector assessment, the extent of need and possible alternatives to residential care were not considered. By the very nature of the private sector of residential care operating as individual units in competition, neither was there any attempt to match individual need to an appropriate setting in order to ensure that needs were met.

Home owners with a preference for people with particular sources of funding. A number of financial sources were identified in the study, ranging from the individual's own capital assets to the state financing of a placement and these are displayed in Table 4.6.

Four homes strongly rejected elderly people who were dependent upon DHSS funding because such residents were likely to be a 'different class of person' or because the owner felt that DHSS funding was set at too low a level to provide 'adequate' care:

> DHSS people aren't in our class. We only admit those with status and wealth and I don't like DHSS people as they are always working class and don't mix well. (The Grange)

> DHSS people are thorns in our side. (Greenfields)

> We'll not take DHSS as the maximum limits set are so ridiculous and I'm worried about who will top up...You can only cater for those on DHSS if you're running a hotel where everyone is mobile. (Elizabeth House)

No home owner appeared to be financially dependent upon DHSS sponsorship and many preferred to have residents with a mix of funding sources. In two homes, DHSS-supported residents paid less than the fees required because the owners had ignored the changing DHSS financial ceiling when introduced in November 1985:

> We've still kept those who've spilt over from the time when DHSS payed full whack. (The Lawns)

This situation, however, can only be sustained in the short-term: with increasing time the DHSS level of funding has not kept pace with fees charged and in order to sustain the business the subsidizing of resident places has diminished.

Another long-established home owner (Underwood), who had no great capital outlay or mortgage to repay and was sufficiently well-off financially, was happy to charge less for DHSS people. In such instances, residents who were self-financing supplemented the home owner's income from DHSS residents.

The attitude of the home owner to the source of funding potentially acted as a barrier to a DHSS recipient. Although few home owners displayed particular attitudes, their charges naturally excluded those on supplementary benefit, unless residents or relatives could guarantee a 'top-up' from other sources.

Fees set by private home owners, particularly in relation to DHSS limits acted as a selectivity point. Nineteen homes (49 per cent) operated an instant bar to those on state funding by setting their fees higher than £125 per week (the Summer 1986 level of DHSS payments). The average fees charged were £126.80 (£1.80 above DHSS limit) which meant that many were only able to become residents via some topping up, via attendance allowance or through other sources of 'goodwill'. The source of extra cash was often unknown to the home owner. Seven homes in the study had evidence of topping up, but another five homes knew very little about the residents' source of funding:

> I get very embarrassed asking about finances - I think most are controlled by the families. (Fenlands)

The average fee of £125 per week, however, disguised the broad range charged by individual homes which varied from £95 to £200 per week (The

Dingle).

Were those residents on DHSS assistance receiving a different service to those *who were self-funding?* Fourteen homes (36 per cent) offered people sponsored by the state a differential service. Unless relatives or 'other parties' topped up, those people on DHSS experienced:

a) A lack of privacy - some residents had to share a double or three-bedded room:

> When the DHSS clamped down we had to juggle rooms around and put DHSS people in double rooms. (Homeview)

Eleven homes offered a premium for a single room.

b) In two homes residents were deprived of extra care and were required to move out if this was necessary.

The majority of home owners said they did not discriminate against state-funded residents or treat them differently, yet the above shows that a minority were discriminating in terms of the provision offered. Choice of extras was sometimes only a reality to those who could afford to pay. Extra payments sometimes guaranteed more personal care (3 homes) and en-suite facilities (6 homes). The differential in fees for such 'luxuries' ranged from £5 to £75, the latter for a single room compared to a double room in one home.

The physical and mental health of elderly people were also significant factors in the selection of residents.

Health factors

The thirty nine homes were ranked on a three point scale according to how important the home owners rated physical and mental health factors in their assessment. Diagram 7.2 shows the main outcomes on the dependency scale.

Mobility. Diagram A shows that home owners said they catered for a range of residents with different mobility levels - for those residents in wheelchairs and those who were fully mobile.

Daily living skills. This factor was divided on the basis of ability to carry out particular tasks. At one extreme, home owners said they accepted residents unable to do three or more tasks (35 per cent) or those who needed twenty four hour care: the mid-range indicated residents who could wash and dress themselves (18 per cent), and the other extreme represented home owners who only accepted residents who were fully independent. A slight skew indicated that a number of homes catered for the marginally more independent in terms of daily living skills (47 per cent).

Continence. A right-hand skew indicated a preference amongst home owners to admit those residents who were fully continent. The thirteen home owners (33 per cent) who admitted incontinent applicants said they had developed coping strategies to accommodate this 'problem'.

Mental state - confusion. The outcome on this measure indicated that a number of homes specialised in the admission of people suffering from senile dementia, while other homes categorically rejected all confused applicants. A further measure of mental state was reflected in the consideration of a person's *psychiatric history.* Most homes (27) assessing for this refused access to anyone with behavioral difficulties or a known psychiatric history. Again, nine homes (23 per cent) accommodating residents with a psychiatric history also accepted confused residents.

Diagram 7.3 represents the findings and shows the variety of provision in the private residential sector. Home owners saw themselves catering across the board for a range of disabilities, physical and mental dependencies, giving variety and choice to a range of people. In this way the finding portrays the unique marketable quality of this sector. At one extreme, homes catered for a heavily dependent population, for example, elderly mentally infirm residents (EMI) who were incontinent, while at the other extreme, a hotel-type model accepted the fit and fully independent clientele.

The middle range of fourteen homes (36 per cent) exhibited a mixture of the two extremes. These homes were further broken down under three main groupings.

1. Two home owners specialised in accommodating elderly mentally infirm people. Very confused and aggressive people were accepted because of the interest, past experience and expertise of the home owners with this group of people. Although both accepted residents with a high level of confusion within the home, one hotel owner rejected people who suffered from incontinence; the other rejected very physically dependent residents, although incontinence was seen as an inevitable consequence of a confusional state.

2. The second group consisted of home owners who accommodated residents with low mobility/daily living skills scores, but high confusion/continence scores. This meant that they did not accept residents who were confused or incontinent but did accept a resident who had a high physical dependency, for example, someone in a wheelchair. Six homes fell into this category. The variation was due to two factors.

DIAGRAM 7.2
LEVELS OF PHYSICAL AND MENTAL DEPENDENCY OF RESIDENTS ACCEPTABLE TO PRIVATE HOME OWNERS

DIAGRAM 7.2A PHYSICAL & MENTAL DEPENDENCY ACCEPTED BY PRIV. HOME OWNERS

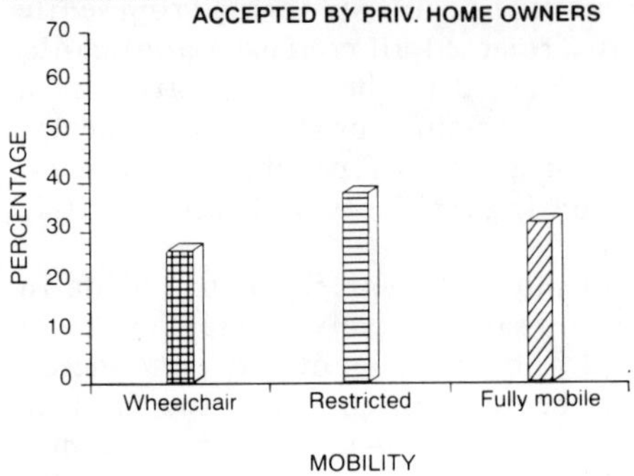

DIAGRAM 7.2B PHYSICAL & MENTAL DEPENDENCY ACCEPTED BY PRIV. HOME OWNERS

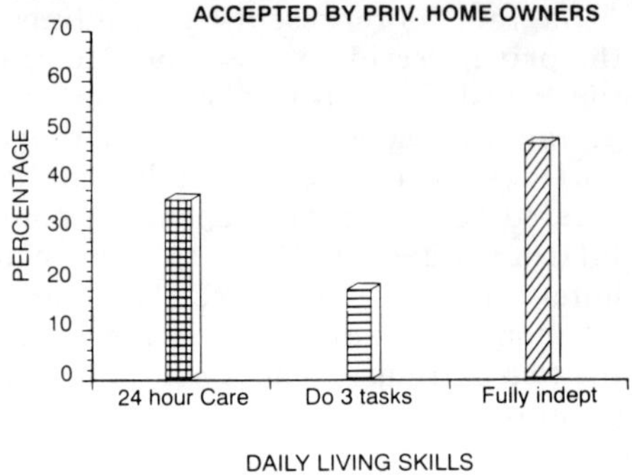

DIAGRAM 7.2C PHYSICAL & MENTAL DEPENDENCY ACCEPTED BY PRIV. HOME OWNERS

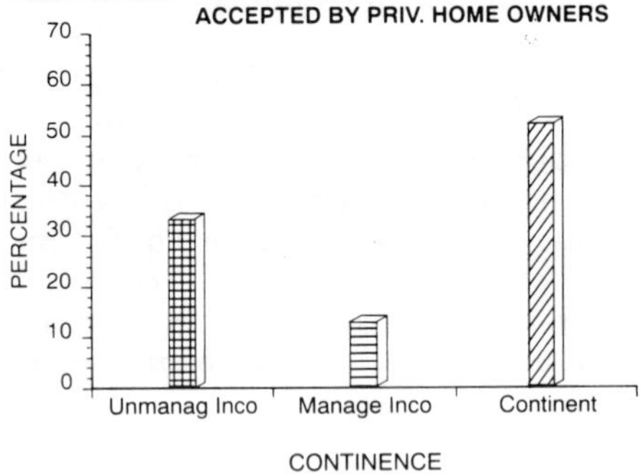

DIAGRAM 7.2D PHYSICAL & MENTAL DEPENDENCY ACCEPTED BY PRIV. HOME OWNERS

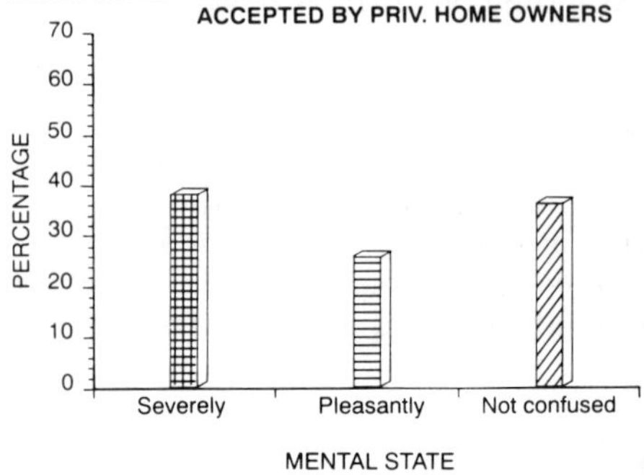

DIAGRAM 7.2E PHYSICAL & MENTAL DEPENDENCY ACCEPTED BY PRIV. HOME OWNERS

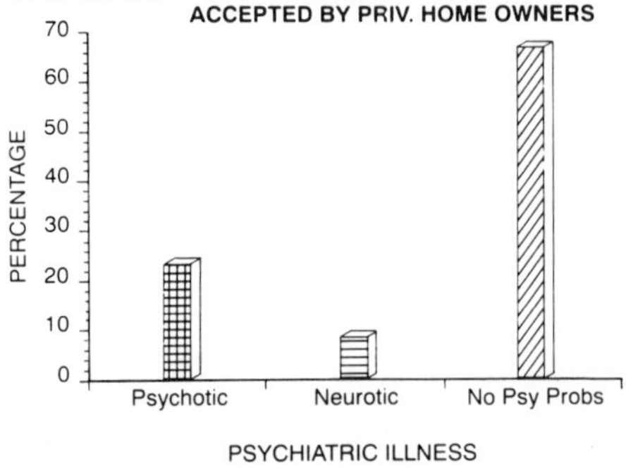

N = 39

DIAGRAM 7.3
AMALGAMATED SCORES FOR ACCEPTED LEVEL OF DEPENDENCY

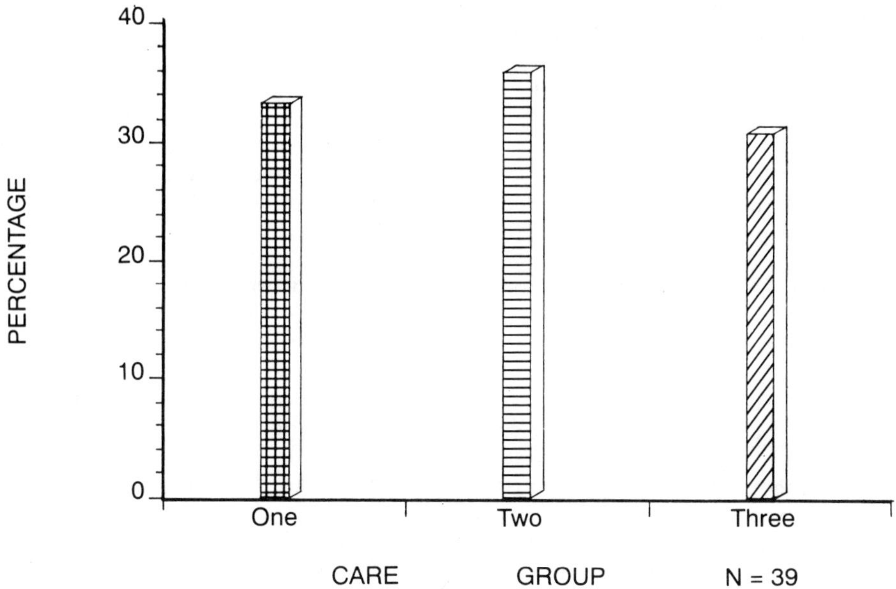

Homes which accept —

Group 1: (scores 4 - 6)	heavy care	residents who were incontinent, wheelchair bound, severely confused and required 24 hours care
Group 2: (scores 7 - 9)	medium care	residents who could wash, dress, carry out 3+ tasks but who had restricted mobility, manageable incontinence or were slightly confused
Group 3 (scores 10 and above)	light care	fully independent, fully continent residents who were not confused

(a) The home owner had either adopted a coping strategy, the environment being adapted to cater for people in wheelchairs or the owner had moved into a purpose-built establishment (2 homes):

> We don't take anyone suffering from senile dementia as it upsets the rest of the home, particularly if they are incontinent, but we're geared up for wheelchair cases. (Millbank)

(b) In other examples, both the home owner and staff were able to manage people in wheelchairs because of their own prior experience and training. One home owner (The Dingle) set its fees higher in order to employ specialist staff. However, the opposite was true in some cases where home owners rejected incontinent people because of the lack of adequate staff to cope with the problem.

3. Other home owners accommodated a variety of people irrespective of their physical and mental condition. These owners did not employ a general policy with regard to admission but assessed each individual 'on their merits':

> We will admit and offer what a caring family should - we set our limits by that - it could include caring for everything. (Inglenook)

A further vital distinction existed between the care groups outlined. Group 1 (heavy end) represented features of a situation akin to a nursing home rather than a residential home (in light of the definition in Home Life, Avebury, 1984). In practice, such a distinction between a nursing and residential home was often blurred with many owners openly acknowledging the nursing care they provided for residents. One home owner felt her marketability and credibility to residents and their relatives was reduced by the fact that she could not advertise as a nursing home as, in all respects, her job was one of providing nursing care. Other home owners felt that caring to the same extent as an ordinary family necessitated some nursing input.

The dividing line between residential and nursing home applicants was, therefore, not clear cut and reflected in a sense the medical ethos adopted by a number of homes and the prevalence and primacy of medical factors in the assessment process.

The emphasis on medical factors in assessment was paramount within the process employed by the majority of home owners. Many included formal admission sheets with details of medical history, diagnoses and bodily function records in their assessment. In twenty eight homes (72 per cent) the main assessment was based on medical factors, very often rejecting at enquiry stage those applicants who did not match the expectation of the home owner:

> If they aren't fit enough, ie. fully independent, we reject at source. (The Rectory)

Social factors

Home owners also based their assessment on the prospective resident's sociability with others, their religious persuasion and social class. Following the medical assessment, the sociability of a resident was important in an acceptance or a rejection. This assessment was again undertaken by the home owner, very often during the resident's day visit or trial period in the home when the home owner observed the elderly person with other residents. Many owners felt that a balance of residents of like mind and behaviour was necessary to the successful and smooth operation of the business.

Religious persuasion was important in three homes (8 per cent) where a Christian ethos was paramount in the philosophy of care (Eastcliffe, The Rest and Inglenook). Owners of these homes believed residents without a religious background would not be comfortable with the routine of daily prayers employed in the home.

Social class featured prominently for two home owners (5 per cent) who assessed for this in the initial enquiry. One only admitted 'gentlefolk' coming from a background with status and wealth:

> If people aren't used to being waited upon, then they don't fit in. (The Grange)

Conclusion

The success or otherwise of securing a private residential home placement depended on getting through various stages in the admission process: processes which were designed and operated by the majority of the thirty nine home owners. The people most likely to complete the process and so gain admission were those who were self-funding and not confused.

Chapter Three described how home owners coming from different backgrounds and operating different philosophies of care within their homes saw themselves offering a varied and credible alternative to local authority provision. Through this variety the private residential sector has developed a unique position in the welfare spectrum. Its main marketing feature is the degree of choice and flexibility that it gives to the individual prospective resident, along with its promotion of independence and status.

However, although home owners saw themselves offering a variety of provision to a number of different people with differing levels of ability, a totally free market did not operate. This was not only because elderly people could not easily select between a variety of alternatives (Chapter Six) but also because the home owner operated restrictive practices in their assessment of the suitability of an elderly person for their home.

A close look at the home owners' policies and practices for admission show restricted choice through the physical, mental and social assessment of prospective residents. Not only did the ability to pay determine the success or rejection of an application but a range of other diverse factors were considered, reflecting the home owners' ability to care for particular residents. Home owners, therefore, distorted the market by operating restrictive practices based on the medical and social assessment of potential residents.

The balance of power in selecting or rejecting residents, extending or restricting choice for particular elderly people remained firmly in the hands of the owner or manager. The demand for a place was such that home owners could be selective.

Most home owners operated very careful selection procedures. There was little evidence of them taking 'anybody' or accommodating only the very fit, independent and lucid resident. In the majority of cases, home owners accepted residents who required the level of care they knew they could give because of their previous experience.

At the end of the day, every home owner had to balance the books and, at least, break even. Consequently the ability to pay was a critical determining factor. Because of this 'choice' was restricted for residents wishing to seek placements in nearly half of the homes (49 per cent) in the study, purely because they were also in receipt of state funding. Even in some of the other twenty homes, where state-supported residents gained entry, they were often faced with a different level of service to those who were self-funding. The 'real' choice of home and care services, therefore, existed for those who were able to pay themselves.

This presents a bleak picture for those who sought a placement and were reliant on state funding. It points to an increasing financial crisis in residential care in the near future as the gap widens between private home fees and the amount the DHSS are prepared to pay. Those who are unable to pay will be forced out of the market unless they can find other means of 'topping up'. This may again place elderly people in a dependent relationship with family members who will have the burden of finding extra sources of funding. In this study only 4 per cent of residents received any extra financial support from their relatives. Although this figure is very low in comparison to the 35 per cent quoted in another recent study (Bradshaw and Gibbs, 1987b), it is not surprising in the context of this study. The figure is an underestimation and not representative of those receiving 'top up' in private care because the study only looked at residents who were in their first year of admission, the majority of whom had previously enjoyed home ownership. As most people were widowed and had no spouse to support, they were able to pay for their care through the sale of their house. The consequences for those residents without additional capital assets when such funding dwindles are yet to be felt in the private sector on a large scale, although recent documentary evidence suggests that residents are beginning to struggle financially in certain parts of the country ('*Who will feed us*? ', Panorama, BBC, 20 February 1989).

Although bureaucratic hurdles were less in private care than in the public sector, other barriers to admission were created by other operators in the process by home owners basing their criteria less on need and more on ability to pay and (as Chapter Eight argues) by social workers refusing to work with the private sector.

8 Key operators in the process of admission: relatives and professionals

The previous chapters show how the operation of the free market cannot easily be applied to the private residential care sector. Prospective residents are unable to choose between a variety of different homes because of their physical or mental state and because of the home owners' restrictive practices.

Chapter Six also demonstrated that relatives are more influential in the process than the prospective resident particularly when it comes to a choice between public and private sectors. This chapter explores further the contribution of relatives and professionals to the process of admission. During the course of the chapter, it will be shown that elderly people and their families choose to ignore the professional's assessment, with relatives taking over the social work role in arranging an admission into private residential care.

Relatives enter the scene mainly as carers, supporting elderly people to remain at home prior to the breakdown of such caring networks which often trigger the process of admission. Elderly people are 'dependent' upon their relatives not only for continuing support at home but also for guidance through the process itself. As this chapter shows, relatives are the major operators directing and influencing the process of decision-making.

In comparison to the influence of relatives, professionals have a marginal role in the process. Although traditionally seen as key operators in admissions to local authority residential homes, the role of the social worker is distorted in the private sector through the operation of market processes; through their own values and political belief systems and the manner in which they perceive their professional role. This renders them less influential in admission to private homes than to local authority homes.

Realistically, choice is limited for elderly people with particular disabilities, such as senile dementia. Elderly people are not empowered by the process to exercise any degree of choice, and even where they have all their faculties, other operators in the process often decide what is best for them.

TABLE 8.1
SIGNIFICANT 'OTHERS' IN THE PROCESS OF ADMISSION

	Private		Local Authority	
	No.	%	No.	%
Son/daughter	88	44	35	29
Other relative	32	16	17	14
Social worker	71	35	120	100
GP/DN/HV/CPN	31	15	11	9
No-one	22	11	0	0
Friend/neighbour	10	5	2	2
Home owner	10	5	0	0
Other	12	6	2	2
[Total no. of residents =	200		120	

Relatives were a major group of people involved in the process of admission into private residential care. Over half (60 per cent) the elderly people who entered a private home involved a relative in some way. A third of private sector residents entered with the help of a social work professional. Less came through health professionals. A small group of twenty two people entered independently of others and could be described as the 'true consumers'.

Relatives as key operators in the process of admission into private residential care

Table 8.1 shows that 60 per cent of elderly people entered private residential care with help from relatives, mainly offspring (44 per cent). Less than half (43 per cent) the elderly people who entered local authority homes involved significant relatives in their admission process. The role of relatives and informal contacts (65 per cent) was greater than the role of professionals (50 per cent).

This section looks at the role of relatives in terms of their involvement and influence in the process of admission. Under what circumstances were they involved in the process of admission into private care?

The relative as carer

One hundred and eight elderly people who identified significant family members involved in their admission described the role of the relative as the primary carer involved in looking after them.

A profile of the carers

a) Relationship to elderly person

The majority of carers were daughters (54 per cent) although wives (6 per cent) and nieces (25 per cent) also provided vital tending and care. Of the male carers, the majority were sons (34 of the 42). The rest were made up of sisters, daughters-in-law and, in one instance, a female cousin. The traditional female role as carer was, therefore, supported by this evidence confirming Finch and Groves' (1980) conclusion that care by the family equates with care by women.

Offspring were significantly involved where the elderly person lived with them, but were less involved where there were elderly married couples caring for each other. Of those married, only 28 per cent involved their offspring in the admission.

b) Age

Table 8.2 shows the age profile of carers. The majority (75 per cent) were approaching or were of retirement age themselves. The 26 per cent over 70 were spouses caring for their partners.

TABLE 8.2
AGE PROFILE OF CARERS

	No.	%
under 40 years	10	9
41 - 50	17	16
51 - 60	29	27
61 - 70	24	22
over 70 years	28	26
	108	100

With the majority of carers (77 per cent) being married, only a small number (24) cared single-handed for their elderly relative. This figure, however, may underestimate the strain which is placed on individual carers in the partnership. It is important to note that those people coming up to retirement age were taking on extra responsibility and in some cases coped with high levels of dependency at a time of life when they could be free of responsibilities, their grown-up children having left the household.

Nature of the caring task (see chapter five). The nature and level of support was not investigated in depth during interviews with residents but relatives were asked how they supported their elderly person. Both personal and practical tasks were mentioned - ranging from getting the elderly person up in the morning, bathing them, cooking, washing clothes, gardening to 'being neighbourly', which meant 'keeping them company and chatting'. Through such efforts, relatives allowed many elderly people to remain in their own homes.

The level of care required by some elderly people and the time necessary for the caring process restricted the life of many carers. Caring for an elderly person became a tie for a number of people and life for some lost spontaneity and vitality. One carer stated:

> I couldn't go out or follow my profession.

Even on a day-to-day basis, some people were constrained. In another example, one daughter talking about her commitment to her mother who had senile dementia, said:

> I couldn't leave her, even for two hours (Daughter of Mrs Dowsing, The Lodge).

Other examples were found where daughters visited their elderly parent up to six times a day. As shown in Chapter Six, some relatives (13) tended more than one dependent person - sometimes their spouse's parents or their own disabled husbands. Carers were sometimes ill themselves (9) or disabled through strokes, angina, arthritis, diabetes and poor mobility. Others suffered nervous breakdowns and received out-patient treatment for depression as a result of the caring task.

One of the significant arenas effected by caring was employment which was often restricted by the commitment to an elderly relative. A daughter commented:

> One couldn't give full support to any elderly person if one is in full-time work.

Another son (of Mrs Pinker, The Lodge) gave up his work as a long-distance lorry driver to care for his confused mother. Others were taking part-time employment:

> As far as employment was concerned I could only take a part-time job.

> Looking after her (mother) was full-time employment.

On the other hand a few people felt their work provided them with an escape from the daily routine of tending:

> Going to work made me think my problem wasn't so bad. I didn't want to give up work. (Daughter of Mrs Drutte, The Dell)

Six examples were found of tension between family members, when living in the same household. Two elderly people described as 'cantankerous', 'manipulative and domineering' and 'demanding' by their relatives had recently entered a private home.

Friction between members was sometimes fuelled through personality clashes; elderly people's feelings of being a burden and, in two cases, accusations made about certain members of the family, led to what one person described as 'civil war'.

In several cases marital difficulties resulted as a consequence of living a fragmented family life:

> For ages my husband and I couldn't go out together as it wasn't safe to leave her - we had no life together. (Daughter of Mrs Gates, Eaton Lodge)

> I was unaware my own life was cracking up. (Daughter of Mrs Doyle, The Lodge)

> I was getting lower - just spending more and more time with her and I didn't have any home life. I had to realise she was not the same friend and let go.

Daughters sometimes expressed difficulty in relation to the role reversal they faced, particularly in caring for fathers who needed personal assistance.

Others took on new roles. A nephew of Mrs Delves (Condor House) tried to carry on where his mother, caring for her brother, had left off prior to her death. With his own disability through a stroke he found this impossible.

Although relatives were not unwilling to take on the caring role, families, and particularly sole carers within the family, found difficulty looking after their elderly relatives. Twenty one per cent of elderly people entered care directly as a result of the family's inability to continue in this role.

Relatives as initiators of the process

There was some evidence that relatives encouraged people to enter residential care because they felt they would be better off. Thirty two examples were found of this. The statement 'she can't cope' was often voiced by relatives, particularly if the elderly person lived alone and had difficulty in managing an independent lifestyle. Anxieties about elderly people placing themselves at risk by leaving on the gas or cooker ran high. For example:

> My nieces are the only ones ever involved. They know what is best. (Mrs Govan, The Limes)

> We persuaded her to go into a private home. I'm now insisting on a single room for her as I know it's best. (niece)

> Just felt mother couldn't look after herself so I brought her. (Son of Mrs Swan, Fairlawns)

We felt she needed care and attention and told her we could arrange it all. (daughter-in-law of Mrs Peters, Fenlands)

Pressure to enter a home was sometimes exerted by relatives to relieve their own anxieties about their isolated and lonely relation:

I persuaded her to go into a home as I was moving and I wanted her settled somewhere before I went. (daughter-in-law of Mrs Crisp, Elizabeth House)

Relatives were also involved where elderly people had previously been in other residential institutions (10 per cent). One relative said: 'we didn't like the new matron so we moved her'.

The relative as decision-maker

Some people took fundamental decisions about moving their elderly relative into residential care.

Table 8.3 illustrates that relatives, in relation to other groups involved with elderly people, were primary decision makers in the process to enter private residential care. Residents and relatives involved in admissions to the private sector had far more 'say' in decision-making than residents and relatives involved in local authority admissions.

TABLE 8.3
WHOSE DECISION TO ENTER RESIDENTIAL CARE?

	Private		Local Authority	
	No.	%	No.	%
Relative	75	38	26	22
Resident	57	28	18	15
Professional	38	19	36	30
Other (including joint decisions)	30	15	40	33
	200	100	120	100

Under what circumstances were relatives taking decisions?
1. Living with other family members became a vulnerable and a potentially insecure setting, with a number of elderly people finding themselves at the will of their relatives. However, for those people living alone or as husband and wife, there was evidence of consultation and a joint decision-making process. Thirty people (57 per cent living in settings other than their 'own home') entered private residential care due to the decision of their relatives.

2. Where elderly people suffered from senile dementia, decisions on future care were taken by relatives. Not surprisingly, people who were confused were unable to make such decisions, this task therefore being abrogated to relatives (see Chapter Five).

3. Thirty one percent of relatives' decisions were taken after a bereavement within the family. This illustrated a particularly vulnerable period for elderly people who very often, after a time of loss, felt incapable of taking future decisions. There was evidence to suggest that relatives played a major role on these occasions:

> It was the shock of her husband dying. At first we felt she could stay at home, but it got too much so we looked for a home. (Relative of Mrs White, Inglenook)

4. Of relatives taking decisions on behalf of elderly people, twenty six (35 per cent) specifically decided on private residential care because they were unable to continue caring. This differed significantly from decisions made by *residents* to enter care because their families were unable (7 per cent).

5. Alongside this, 57 per cent of relatives' decisions came as a result of pressure being exerted on the resident and family from a number of sources i.e. doctors, other professionals and neighbours all pushing for 'something' to be done. A few families themselves pressurized the elderly person, to the extent that some felt powerless and helpless to argue against the decision:

> If they said it was OK I fitted in. I wasn't in a position to argue with all their decisions. (Miss Elliot, The Yarmouth)

> My daughter just put it to me one day - we've got a nice home for you to go to. (Mr Kirk, The Dingle)

Some decisions made by relatives were due to an accumulation of other pressures and were taken out of the elderly person's hands without consultation. The pressure of time led to one relative presenting his confused mother with a fait accompli:

> I decided there and then we should take the vacancy - I'd only been in for a chat but I didn't want to miss the opportunity. (son of Mrs Clinton, Willow House)

Other elderly people were consulted and agreed, but under duress. It was not only a single decision, therefore, taken by a relative that triggered entry into residential care but rather a series of decisions; from a decision by relatives that the elderly person could not cope alone or the family could not continue their support, to the decision that a private residential home placement was the best option.

Relatives were not only influential in persuading elderly people that residential care would be best for them, they were also primary influences in the decision-making process and as Chapter Six showed, in finding a suitable private home.

The relative as selector. Relatives were also instrumental in looking around and choosing the home suitable for the elderly person. Some phoned a series of homes and took the first vacancy, while others carefully planned and scrutinized a number of homes before deciding between a range of options:

> I was instrumental in phoning and took the first vacancy. (Relative of Mr Crossland, Seaview)

> I got a list and phoned sixteen places and went around them all. (Relative of Mrs York, The Suffolk)

Even in situations where the elderly person decided on residential care, the initial search for a home was often undertaken by a relative with a limited choice presented to the elderly person; relatives decided on the more suitable residential accommodation and very often drew up a short list of homes, based on the location, size and atmosphere (Chapter Six).

Relatives were also influential in negotiating the placement on the elderly person's behalf with the home owner and in six cases negotiating financial arrangements with the DHSS, the latter often after admission.

Twelve instances were found where elderly people accepted vacancies prior to any visit or inspection of the home:

> My niece came to have a look; she said it was a nice place - I didn't even visit. (Mrs Leyman, The Yarmouth)

> We went to see her after we'd placed her there and then had to negotiate to get her out as she wasn't happy. (Relative of Mrs Thomas, The Orchard)

In this case, the home owner discouraged relatives from visiting during the trial month, to enable the resident to settle. Even where residents had the opportunity to view private homes, only nineteen enjoyed the benefit of a short-term stay in the home prior to admission.

Although no questions were asked relating to the continuing involvement of relatives once the elderly person was in a home, some residents freely commented on how their relative supported them after their admission, for example through visiting, selling their house and dealing with financial affairs.

The role of relatives in the process of admission

1. Relatives were involved in the admission of elderly people to private homes and were major decision makers in the process, particularly if the elderly person lived alone, with relatives or in another residential setting, if they suffered from senile dementia and if the family found they were unable to continue caring.

2. There was evidence to support the proposition that relatives influenced

elderly people in their decision to enter private homes because they thought they would be better off. However, there was no evidence that relatives were unwilling to care, or of widespread conflict between relatives and residents and little evidence that relatives pushed their elderly folk against their will, although elderly people were found to be compliant with their wishes.

3. Relatives took the primary role in the direction and management of the process. In a number of cases the family's inability to continue caring initiated the process of admission. When they were unable to care they looked to the commercial residential sector for relief: for them, the private residential sector was more flexible and available at the crucial time. The features found in private homes - such as privacy and security - attracted relatives.

The ideology of the free market allows, in theory, for freedom of choice to the individual but this choice is dependent on the knowledge and availability of alternatives (Chapter Six). However, where there was a degree of choice, it was available to the relative. Relatives decided not only on residential care, but on the suitability of the home, and negotiated the process of admission, usually alongside the elderly person.

4. Relatives were also the major stakeholders in the admission of elderly people into residential care. Many gained peace of mind by persuading the elderly person to enter a private home. Others were able to return to full-time employment. Relatives' influence, however, may have different consequences for the resident. It creates dependency which may not only extend through the process but also be taken into residential life within the home. The elderly person's quality of life may suffer as they perceive themselves in a dependent role, leaving decision-making to others. Also what suits a relative may not suit the resident. Relatives, in selecting a suitable home, looked for different things to residents. Security, for example, was more important to relatives, whereas most residents wanted more independence and consequently more risk taking.

Relatives were empowered in the process of admission to private residential care unlike the process of admission into local authority residential care where a professional assessment of their role and influence took place. One consequence of a professional assessment in the private sector would be, therefore, to force families to care within a community setting, particularly if residential resources are scarce.

Role of the social worker in admission to private residential care

Phillips and Vincent (1986b) found the most significant channel into private homes in Devon was through contact with a social worker. They show that almost seventy five per cent of homes received one of their five most recent residents through an introduction from a social worker. They go on to say:

> The implications of the importance of social workers as a first contact are considerable as these people will be able to exercise choice and

professional judgement about the suitability of any particular homes for specific residents. (Phillips & Vincent, 1986 p.166)

The traditional role and skills exercised by a social worker in a professional assessment of elderly people seeking residential care have been extended to the private sector over a number of years. Little research has been carried out, however, on the actual role they perform and the status they hold within the market system.

The reactions of social workers to private sector growth and increased responsibility placed upon such public agents to help elderly people in the journey into a competing sector of care is analysed in this section. It attempts to investigate five areas:

1. Under what circumstances did social workers direct people to the private sector?

2. What kind of social workers advocated private care in preference to a public care system?

3. What role social workers performed in private sector admissions.

4. How much influence they held in a competing sector of care.

5. What implications there are of increased social work activity in the private sector.

Methodology and analysis

Social workers, identified by elderly residents as significant in their process of admission, were interviewed using an interview checklist. This was designed to identify the social worker and their place of work; to give information regarding their involvement in the admission of a specific individual to private residential care; to examine their perception of the role played by relatives and other professionals in the process and to look at their attitudes towards the private sector.

In addition to this, a range of material was collected from residents and their relatives reflecting their experiences of social workers in the process of admission.

Two groups of social workers, one in the private sector, the other in the public sector, were identified. The first group (42) were involved in some respect with an actual admission into private care: the second group (50) placed an elderly person in a local authority home and in contrast were not necessarily involved with placements in the private sector.

There were certain advantages in using two 'groups' of social workers:

1. There were a number of similarities between the groups. They were in touch with similar people in the population and, secondly, they worked for the same local authority and therefore worked under the same overall policy, agency philosophy and practice guidelines in relation to elderly people and the private sector.

2. Twelve social workers who were interviewed were common to both groups, suggesting some measure of overlap between the two groups.

3. A range of social work views were represented.

The extent to which social workers were involved in the private sector compared to the public sector highlighted the different systems in operation and the different processes in admission to the two settings. In other words, in order for an elderly person to gain entry to a local authority home, a social worker was obliged to assess their need for residential provision. Engaging a social worker to help in admission to private care in many cases was a discretionary choice exercised by elderly people themselves or their families.

In the analysis of the data, it was therefore difficult to directly compare the two sectors in terms of those who did and those who did not have a social worker, as all admissions to public care involved the social worker in the capacity of assessor and gatekeeper to resources. The descriptions and case studies illustrated in this section therefore refer to the private sector alone; the local authority material is used for comparative purposes where possible.

Profile of social workers

Forty two social workers were interviewed in relation to their role and involvement in 71 admissions into private residential care (group 1). Twelve of these social workers were again interviewed in the study of local authority admissions (group 2). In this latter survey, fifty social workers (38 of whom were different from the social workers interviewed in group 1) were interviewed in depth regarding both their role relating to 113 cases in admission to local authority residential care and attitude toward participation in admissions to private homes. In total, the views of 80 (42 + 50 - 12) social workers were represented in this material.

The majority of social workers were female (74 per cent). No additional information on age, marital status, training or years of experience was gained consistently but, from retrospective analysis, social workers in the total sample of eighty tended to be qualified social workers (52 per cent) and social work assistants (14 per cent). [The remaining 34 per cent had left the department and details of their qualifications were not available.]

Those involved in private sector admissions (Group 1). Eighteen (43 per cent) social workers were located in area offices in the county and were involved mainly with admissions directly from the community which they served. Twenty four social workers in the private sector study (57 per cent) were hospital based: 17 (40 per cent) from a general hospital and 7 (17 per cent) from a psychiatric hospital.

Such numbers reflected the fact that social workers were more likely to help people who were in hospital (53 per cent) than those coming from home where a relative was more important in arranging the admission. This was not surprising as elderly people were more likely to meet a social worker if coming from a setting in which other professionals were involved in their care and where different circumstances surrounded the process of admission (ie, they lived alone and were unsupported by formal services).

TABLE 8.4
SIGNIFICANT 'OTHERS' IN ADMISSION TO PRIVATE HOMES AND RESIDENTS' SOURCE OF ADMISSION

	Relatives		Social workers		Others	
	No.	%	No.	%	No.	%
Hospital	40	35	38	53	39	42
Home	43	37	19	27	47	50
Other	32	28	14	20	7	8
	115	100	71	100	93	100

Profile of elderly people engaging a social worker

As Table 8.1 shows, 35 per cent of elderly people (71) who entered private residential care involved a social worker in their admission. Social workers took a back seat in contrast to relatives, but were more significant in numbers than other professionals in the process of admission.

Social workers worked with a cross section of elderly people who entered private residential care under a variety of circumstances: not only those people who lived alone or who 'needed' care and residential support, but a range of 'independent' people in the community were guided by a social worker into a private home.

A considerable part of social work activity, however, in the private sector was spent in the admission of those people who were confused (60 per cent of social work activity involved work with confused people) and who entered residential care when family networks and supports withdrew through their inability to continue caring (48 per cent).

Social workers were equally engaged in both crisis and planned admissions into private care but a greater percentage of crisis admissions involved social workers (55 per cent) than planned admissions (27 per cent).

A further examination, therefore, was made of the circumstances under which social workers were involved in the admission. The choice to engage a social worker in the process of admission did not totally lie in the hand of the elderly client or consumer - the entry into a private home via a social work professional depended partly on the relatives decision as to whether a social worker was necessary and the personal value system of the social worker and circumstances that he or she weighed up in coming to a decision to become involved in the process of admission.

Participation of social workers in the private sector

The two groups of social workers interviewed, one involved in private sector admissions, the other with local authority residents, gave a variety of reasons why they were involved in admissions to private sector homes. In some cases the decision was taken on the basis of their personal and political values relating to private care, and how they perceived their role within the agency

- as gatekeepers and catalysts for resources within the public sector alone, or as advocates on behalf of their clients irrespective of the sector within which they operated.

Circumstances at a particular time also influenced participation; for example, a lack of local authority resources forced a pragmatic move to the private sector; in circumstances where an elderly person lacked family members who could petition and negotiate entry into care on their behalf, some social workers fulfilled what was seen by other social workers to be the relatives' responsibility in relation to the private sector.

Table 8.5 summarizes the circumstances under which social workers were involved in an admission to the private sector. The first column describes the reasons why 42 social workers participated in admissions to private care in the previous year. Column 2 represents hypothetical circumstances under which the local authority sample of social workers said they would become involved in a private sector admission. The twelve social workers who were also actively engaged in admissions to both private and public homes were excluded from this analysis.

It is interesting to note that 43 per cent of those working with the private sector held politically favourable views towards private care. Interviews with social workers who placed elderly people in local authority homes in the previous year revealed negative views toward privatization. Only four held political preferences for the private sector.

This indicates that there were social workers who were politically in favour of the private system and who directed people into private care.

Of the total sample population of 200, 89 (44 per cent) said they had contact with a social worker in their process of admission. However, 18 people said that the social worker withdrew their services after the initial contact. Although the remaining social workers provided a service to 71 (35 per cent), they did not enjoy a uniform service (Table 8.6). This service ranged from giving elderly people or their relatives a list of homes and a recommendation, to a full assessment and placement service.

The majority of residents (65 per cent) therefore entered private residential care without a social worker (15 per cent involved other professionals who provided an indirect link to a social worker).

TABLE 8.5
CIRCUMSTANCES UNDER WHICH SOCIAL WORKERS WERE INVOLVED IN THE PRIVATE SECTOR

	Private		Local Authority	
	No.	%	No.	%
In the best interests of the elderly person	16	38	5	13
Pragmatic - no public sector resources	17	40	16	42
Political preference for one sector (i.e. private)	18	43	4	10
No family involved	2	5	6	16
Knowledge of homes	10	24	18	47
Number of social workers =	42		38*	

* Excluding 12 in private sector

TABLE 8.6
CIRCUMSTANCES UNDER WHICH ELDERLY PEOPLE DID NOT HAVE A SOCIAL WORKER INVOLVED IN THEIR PRIVATE SECTOR ADMISSION

	Elderly people	
	No.	%
Elderly person did not request a social work service	97	48
Families ignored the existing social work service	6	3
Other professionals bypassed the social work service	8	4
Social workers saw their role purely in the state system	8	4
Social workers withdrew - because of their political values	8	4
Social workers withdrew - because elderly people's families were involved	2	1
	129	65%

Circumstances under which social workers were not involved or withdrew from private care

There were seven main reasons why social workers were not engaged in the process of admission (Table 8.6). Ninety seven elderly people (48 per cent) did not want a social worker involved in their admission or were not aware of the social worker's role in such matters. There was also evidence that families (3 per cent) and other professionals (4 per cent) bypassed the social work service after a social worker was initially involved.

Eight admissions (4 per cent) of elderly people into private care had no involvement with a social worker due to the political views held by the social worker in relation to private care. In a further eight (4 per cent) examples, the social worker saw her role entirely in the public system and withdrew when there were no resources available in this sector or when the elderly person was not eligible for public sector residential care. In two instances in this category, social workers did not transfer their assessment skills to the private sector because they believed the elderly person had enough money and could employ others, such as solicitors to look into this process on their behalf. Social workers in this group saw their role purely for those who could not afford the choice of private care.

Social workers also withdrew where families were on hand to participate in the process of admission (1 per cent). There were few examples, therefore, of social workers who were hostile to and detached from the private sector withdrawing after initial contact and not providing a service.

1. Elderly people did not request a social work service. Ninety seven elderly people entered directly without the involvement of any professional. Elderly people such as these and their families could be described as customers, buying into the private service directly - unlike those who entered a local authority home and were required to go through a social worker's assessment for suitability. The market was flexible to respond to what the customer wanted without the involvement or interference of a social worker.

2. Families ignored the existing social work service. Six families chose to ignore the social worker in the process of admission of their elderly relative. The previous section highlighted relatives as influential agents in the process of admission, holding more knowledge and access to a range of alternatives on which to base a decision than the elderly person and often the social worker.

> I picked up the case when she was admitted to hospital and my main contact was with the son. In discussing future plans we had a chat about homes, particularly local authority residential homes and the waiting list. He agreed to return to me, but never did. (Social worker for Mrs Thomas, The Lawns).

> I was involved in discussing future plans and I assessed her for different options, but they didn't look at any homes with me as the daughter presented it to me *fait accompli* - they had found a vacancy and just put it to me. (Social worker for Mrs Vickery, The Suffolk)

Some families did not find social workers helpful - partly through a lack of clarity in their involvement and because of their lack of knowledge about homes. As a result, many relatives saw no reason to keep social workers informed of their dealings with the private sector.

> I got an appointment with the social worker who I think helped all she could, and was very nice, but she only came once and I can't remember what she suggested. (Daughter of Mrs Chrissian, Limestone)

> We lost the social worker somewhere along the way - I guess she had a large caseload. I don't think she was very good. I don't know what she was trying to do. (niece of Mrs Bott, Fenlands)

Other relatives disliked the 'gatekeeping' function of social workers, seeing them only as gatekeepers to local authority resources, and preferred to have direct involvement with the home owners.

3. Other professionals bypassed the social work service. In eight (4 per cent) admissions of elderly people to residential care, other professionals such as

GPs and CPNs saw the role of the social worker contained within the public sector alone. They saw no reason to involve a social worker in the alternative process of admission to private care, when they could take on the function of negotiating a placement themselves.

A community psychiatric nurse involved in admission of patients from one local psychiatric hospital to a number of private homes, described her view of the process. She believed that social workers were only prepared to consider elderly people 'at risk' which did not include those who had already spent a lengthy period in a long-stay psychiatric hospital. In her eyes, facilitating admission to a local authority residential home was the only 'legitimate' role for social workers and, when this was not under consideration, there was no further role for them. She also believed that there were seldom vacancies where and when they were needed in local authority residential accommodation. Other CPNs at the same hospital felt that they had equally good knowledge of the private residential sector along with an understanding of the needs of elderly people and thus could operate without a social worker as third party in the admission process. Their contact with patients over several years put them in a more favourable position than a social worker coming into the hospital as a stranger to the elderly person.

4. Social workers saw their role purely in the state system. In 4 per cent of admissions of elderly people into the private sector, the social worker withdrew because of the lack of appropriate resources in the public sector. They did not see their role as extending into the private sector.

The influence of the social worker in the process and the extent to which they could offer choice to elderly people was determined in part by the resources available. The lack of resources in the public sector disempowered social workers as primarily public sector agents in the process and as a result they withdrew, seeing themselves in no useful role in an alternative system.

The social worker's role was one of initial assessment and then withdrawal when resources were not available.

> The social worker became involved again when I was in hospital and suggested local authority residential but there weren't any vacancies. That was the end of the social worker. (Mrs Lewis, The Orchard)

> While she was in hospital I made several attempts to rehabilitate her but it was no good. I did try local authority residential but a long-stay placement was virtually impossible so I gave up. (Social worker for Mrs Grove, Underwood)

Elderly people often faced by a 'tramline' response of the social worker were left with no choice or information regarding possible alternatives.

In three cases where elderly people were assessed not eligible for public residential care, social workers did not actively encourage the private sector; they just withdrew. This indicates that they used the same model of assessment across both sectors.

5. *Political values.* There was evidence in the private sector study, relating to 4 per cent of the sample, that social workers were politically opposed to working within the private sector. In such cases the personal values and preferences of social workers acted as barriers to choice for elderly people. This is an interesting figure as it suggests that there were fewer hard line social workers than one might imagine. However, this figure may be an underestimation as some social workers may have deterred people from private care completely and therefore they would not have entered the sample. Other social workers compromised their values with the 'urgency' of finding a residential home.

Several comments from social workers involved in the local authority sector (group 2) mirrored their political preference. One social worker involved with a family considering residential care withdrew when they decided on the private sector:

> I don't want to deal with the private sector. I just will explain about it. It seems unfair that we get these able-bodied and have to help them out, particularly if they can't pay - rather than dealing with the pressing needs in our own homes.

Other social workers held similar views:

> Personally I disapprove. It doesn't offer safeguards, consistency, protection and security. All it does is make profit.

> I don't consider private, due to my own thinking. Ours are better.

> I shy away from the private sector due to my personal policies. I don't favour privatization, and I've resisted the policy moves.

> Politically I don't like them. As a social worker I'm not a political animal.

Five social workers felt that people with money should not block local authority residential provision but exercise their ability to pay for private care: they felt that choice via the ability to pay was something they did not want to be involved with in any way:

> I decided between local authority and private care on a financial basis - people who pay can go their own way.

> People shouldn't necessarily have priority in our homes if they have money.

> If it's urgent and they can afford it I tell them to look to the private sector.

Alternatively, other social workers regarded their primary role in the private sector as one of advising relatives about finance.

6. Social workers withdrew because elderly people's families were involved. Two social workers were not involved in the private sector because of the presence of sons and daughters to help their elderly parents in the process of admission. Social workers often saw families as natural advocates for elderly people whatever circumstances they faced - even if families were unable to continue in a caring role or unwilling to participate in the admission. Some social workers felt the responsibility for the admission should rest with the relatives:

> The social worker was involved following a request for short-term care to cover us while on holiday. Mother's physical and mental state deteriorated while she was in short-term care. My husband refused to have her home. The social worker offered us day care and gave us a list - we had to find a home ourselves. (Daughter of Mrs Selway, The Grange)

> If there are relatives, the most I'll do is give information. I'm a local authority social worker so relatives must deal with the private sector. (Social worker)

Social workers also felt they should not intrude in the private relationship and negotiation between families and home owners:

> If the family are keen on private care after I've explored the option of residential care with them, then they can go away and explore it themselves. We tell them about it but it's a private arrangement. (Social worker)

> The social worker just faded away when we mentioned the private sector. It was right back to us. (Daughter of Mrs Glamorgan, Willow House)

> The social worker left it up to us, with no explanation. She just left it up to us to look for a vacancy. (Relative of Mr Houghton, Greenfields)

Families experiencing these attitudes often felt unsupported and lost and in such cases were forced to be the main motivators in the process. Some held very little knowledge of where to turn next for recommendations and information. The social worker often abrogated their role as advisor and facilitator of residential services to relatives. Relatives were therefore empowered in the process by the transfer and negation of traditional professional roles.

7. Summary of non-involvement. Social workers described in this group were not...

> an independent voice on behalf of the client, enabling the client, as far as possible, to make personal decisions, which might be different from those made by relatives or friends.
> (BASW, 1984, p.9, paragraph 3.3.4)

In some cases social workers presented their own political preferences in favour of preferences of the elderly person, and deprived people of an informed choice by withdrawing from the situation.

A quarter (12) of the social workers in the local authority survey held political views opposing the private sector and refused to work within it. They also were potentially depriving elderly people of choice. Some of their comments were included above.

Circumstances under which social workers were involved in the admission to private care

Table 8.5 shows that some social workers actively participated in the process of admission of elderly people to the private sector. Thirty eight per cent of social workers considered the welfare of elderly people as paramount and worked within the private sector if this furthered their best interests.

Five groups of social workers were identified regarding the reasons they gave for being involved in private sector admissions. Some of these social workers held negative views of the private system seeing it as exploitative but were forced by lack of resources to seek alternative residential provision in the sphere of private welfare (40 per cent). A larger percentage (43 per cent) held favourable political views toward the private sector. Ten (24 per cent) were involved actively over a period of time in which they collected considerable and favourable knowledge about the homes in this sector and placed elderly people in the private sector based on their preference for particular homes.

Two social workers (5 per cent) said they were involved in the admission because there were no relatives or friends to act on the elderly person's behalf.

In the best interest of the elderly person. Social workers were actively involved with private sector admissions because 16 social workers felt it met the needs of the elderly person in the most appropriate way. They held no preference for one sector of care over the other but private care was seen as being the *most appropriate* response in that the home was able to cater for the professionally assessed needs of the elderly person:

> I assessed together with the consultant and we made a conscious decision to place this lady in a Catholic home, it was the best placement as her life style was parallel - this woman had always lived in a convent. The home owner was a Catholic and understood the Catholic culture. The home could also contain her dementia and behaviour difficulties. We therefore opted for this home. (Social worker for Miss Waters, Crabfield)

A pragmatic response. Seventeen (40 per cent) of the 42 social workers working with the private sector expressed mixed feelings about their role and considered themselves forced into accepting their position because of the lack of resources in the public sector. They saw themselves, first and foremost, as gate-keepers to the local authority sector but, when there were no vacant beds in their own homes, or 'waiting lists' were long, they turned to the private sector for help.

A lack of resources steered the social worker into the private sector. The inadequacies of local authority provision included the lack of vacancies, particularly for married couples. For example:

> I had to act fast - they couldn't get a local authority residential placement together so I had to look for a vacancy. There were never two vacancies so I had to look to the private sector. This home could offer a vacancy and the fees were in the DHSS guidelines. (Social worker for Mr and Mrs Sixsmith, The Suffolk)

This next example also highlighted the inflexibility of the public sector to deal with emergency admissions in the same way as the private sector. For example:

> I tried to rehabilitate her home, but her sister withdrew her support and the hospital were pressurizing me to get rid of her - there were no vacancies in local authority residential. (Social worker for Mrs Drew, The Bridges).

> By the time she was prepared to go into a home there weren't any vacancies in local authority residential. I'm afraid I had to use the private system and I phoned to see what vacancies were available. I couldn't get involved in any of the planning and my social work input was inadequate. (Social worker for Mrs Knight, The Orchard)

[A further placement had to be found when Mrs Knight became incontinent.]

This demonstrates just two of the constraints on the social workers in seeking a residential placement in the public sector. Firstly, the constraint of time when local authority vacancies were not instantly available when the client (and sometimes social worker) chooses and, secondly, the lack of resources.

Social workers expressed a variety of personal feelings about being forced into a situation with the private sector because of a lack of places in local authority residential homes. For some social workers a *relationship of necessity* with the private sector was fostered by the lack of appropriate resources in the public sector.

> We are forced to use the private sector a lot. In principle we don't like it. When people can't go home from hospital and have to await a local authority residential vacancy, then it's often the case we have to look to the private sector.

The lack of control over the private sector, not only in relation to standards and variability of provision, but in terms of pace of the admission process and the lack of ability to monitor and review situations after elderly people were placed, left some social workers feeling uncomfortable and in an uneasy relationship with home owners.

Other social workers were more positive about their relationship with the private sector. Although the lack of resources steered them to work with private home owners, they saw this as a positive move and the only way forward:

> Because of the pressure on beds, I use the private sector as much as possible. They are quick and helpful.

A different picture emerged from the general hospital in respect of the social worker's role in the care system. Social workers from the field commented on this:

> Hospital workers seem to take a very different attitude.
>
> The picture is very different from the hospital.

Many hospital social workers felt they were forced to use the private sector because people were otherwise caught between being unable to go home and having to wait for a local authority residential vacancy. Such a wait in hospital often meant blocking the system which aggravated consultants wanting to move people out of hospital.

Under these circumstances, the role of the social worker was different. In some cases their role became 'an administrative one of moving bodies from hospital to private homes', with such social workers seen as 'hand-maidens' of consultants who were 'hot on the idea of private care as it cleared beds quicker than in local authority residential' (field social workers).

Other social workers felt the private sector should only be used if it served individual needs of the client; this often meant taking on the role as advocate/opponent to medical pressure or a buffer position between client/patient and consultant:

> They are wanting people out as soon as possible despite all and expecting us to place them in private homes.

This confirms the findings of Neill (1982) that social workers in a hospital setting face different circumstances surrounding the process of admission than field social workers.

Political preference for the private sector. Eighteen social workers placed elderly people in the private sector because of their political preferences. Although this involved a small number (18) of elderly people out of the total, nearly half (43 per cent) of the social workers interviewed expressed their preference for the private sector over the public sector. The majority of such social workers expressing a preference (52 per cent) worked in a hospital setting. Not only did most feel the private sector relieved the pressure upon them to find placements, but they also felt the sector provided more choice. For example:

> I never pursue local authority residential because of the delay and I always look at the private sector first, it gives people more choice...in terms of size, variety and places.

> Local authority residential is the last resort. I haven't got two years to wait around. You can get a better deal in the private sector. (Social worker for Mr Fox, The Beeches)

The advantage of choice (of home, single room, and timing of admission) was the main political point on which these social workers advocated private care.

Where no family were involved with the elderly person. Two of the forty two social workers (5 per cent) were obliged to use the private sector, acting as advocates on the elderly people's behalf where no family existed to take on the role:

> I leave it to the relatives but if there aren't any relatives, I push myself.

> It all depends on the relatives' presence or absence. I advise them if they are around. If they are absent or incapable, I do all the social work follow-up, even up to one year.

One social worker was reluctant to place those elderly people who were incapable, particularly the elderly mentally infirm, unless relatives were involved.

Knowledge of homes. There was evidence to indicate that some residents were directed into particular private homes because 10 (24 per cent) social workers fostered a good working relationship with the home owner and promoted particular private homes. In other words, social workers knew what the variety of homes in their 'patch' offered. In discussion with the social workers, some saw themselves in the role of investigating the 'good' while boycotting the 'bad' homes and building up links with the 'good' home owners. They therefore extended their role within the private system as monitor, investigator and gatekeeper - seeing their role in building up and fostering relationships in an alternative sector as a legitimate one of a public sector employee:

> I pop in as much as I can when passing.

> I don't know what we'd do without them. I'm very glad they're here. I know all the local homes and I usually use a few private homes that I know well. In fact I visit every week. They sometimes use us as consultants too.

This last statement indicated that the relationship was used to the advantage of home owners as well as social workers. As a result of such positive two-way contact, there was evidence that social workers, particularly hospital based, channelled elderly people into homes with which they had well established links.

Two social workers (one from an area team, one from a general hospital) both directed seven clients to two particular homes where they had successfully placed elderly people over a number of years. In several homes, a group of three residents interviewed came via the same social worker. This indicates that social workers were strongly recommending particular homes.

The community psychiatric nurses who were interviewed also directed elderly patients from a particular hospital setting to certain private homes along what they called a 'classical' route. Channelling between psychiatric hospitals and the specialist private homes for the EMI was evident. The reasons were explained by one social worker:

> The home owner is a trained psychiatric nurse and her husband a former social worker, who provide a very special 'asylum' situation for the extremely difficult cases of confusion. The home is also situated in an area of the country where there are no other facilities for EMI whatsoever.

The evidence above, therefore, indicated that a small number of professionals saw their role in the private sector akin to their role in the local authority sector. They fostered links with certain homes because they knew 'the home owner could handle the elderly patient', they would be given first chance of vacancies arising, and they were able to monitor the 'progress' of the client once in the home.

Summary of those involved. Social workers placing elderly people in private homes were generally in favour of the private sector or felt comfortable working within it. Excluding the twelve social workers who were involved in both studies, those in the local authority survey said they would have placed elderly people in private care less out of political preference (10 per cent) than pragmatic necessity (42 per cent).

The role of the social worker in the private sector

Social workers in the private sector survey were asked what role they fulfilled with regard to each individual case. The description also included the views of clients and relatives.

For 71 (35 per cent) elderly people, the social worker acted in some way to provide a service. The service, however, varied enormously. Some social workers marginally recognised the private sector in their involvement, preferring to work on the fringes of private care by only giving basic information or a list. Some pointed out to families the necessary procedure (for example, to scan through Yellow Pages or recommended a visit to a number of homes prior to a decision), but did not actively engage themselves in the process and withdrew from further involvement leaving the placement negotiation to others, generally relatives. Others participated through the whole process of admission ending in placement and review (12 per cent). Table 8.7 summarises the levels of involvement.

TABLE 8.7
LEVEL OF SOCIAL WORK ACTIVITY IN THE PRIVATE RESIDENTIAL CARE ADMISSION PROCESS

	No. elderly people involved	% total sample (n=200)
Marginal involvement (e.g. list given)	18	9
Recommended a private home, but no follow-up	14	7
Assessed for residential care, but no follow-up	11	5
Assessed, list given and a home recommended	4	2
Full participation - assessment, placement and follow-up	24	12
	71	35

Marginal involvement. Included in this group of eighteen elderly people were those who said they received financial advice and information from their social worker. One social worker reflected this:

> I assist them in finding out about supplementary benefit.

Some social workers issued leaflets relating to standards, answered questions about private homes or even pointed out the advantages and disadvantages of all the particular options available. Even in this sense, by outlining the options and pointing out the implications of each option, social workers made people aware of their choice. Some social workers openly felt their role was one of by informing people of the existence of the private sector. The following comments given by relatives describe this role:

> We contacted social services as part of the way in but there was no involvement apart from a list. (Relative of Mrs Brookman, Conifers)

> The social worker told us that with our financial circumstances we'd be better off in a private home. We never saw him again, but he promised to help if we were stuck. (Relative of Mrs East, The Rectory)

Some social workers provided information and advice because they saw this as a legitimate role and appropriate response and because they believed there was neither further *need* for involvement nor necessity or eligibility on the client's part for a residential placement.

Recommendation, encouragement, persuasion. Seven per cent of elderly people were recommended private homes by social workers. A number of statements made by social workers indicate this:

- We give an indication.
- I'll dissuade them from going into certain homes.
- I suggest a few good ones to relatives.
- I steer them in the best direction.
- I'll say where I've had a satisfactory experience and where not.

Some elderly people were specifically directed to homes in the private sector, more so than in the public sector:

> The social worker recommended this private home to me. I'd been in a local authority home for short-term care, but she said this home was a better option. (Miss Crisse, The Windmill)

Social workers therefore stepped out of their role as local authority agents and actively involved themselves in the private sector.

Social worker as assessor and gatekeeper. Thirty nine elderly people were assessed for residential care and in twenty eight cases, following assessment, they received either a list (2), recommendation (2) or further involvement (24). The remaining eleven people were left without any follow-up.

The social worker's primary role in the public sector with regard to admission was to indicate 'need' for residential care. However, there was no obligation on the social worker to continue after assessment revealed that the elderly person was not in need of residential care. Elderly people and their families also chose at this stage to ignore the social workers' judgement on need and eligibility (based on their experience in relation to local authority homes) and sought a placement in the private sector.

The complexity of the social workers' role in the assessment of need can be seen further here. Some social workers (mainly field social workers) assessed the situation using innovative and imaginative schemes to keep people in the community. When the situation at home broke down, often requiring a short stay in hospital, families often received a different response from social workers. The same field workers were often undermined by other social workers (particularly hospital based) who 'had a lower level of commitment to packages of community care' and directed families and clients to the private sector without assessing their ability to remain in a community setting: in other words, they were seen to be deciding between the private/public option and not a residential/community care option.

Full involvement in the process. Twenty four elderly people (12 per cent) went through the process of admission with the social worker playing a significant part throughout, via assessment, decision-making, providing a choice of home, negotiating the placement, enabling the client through the transition period, and through the practicalities of admission itself. Some went on to support and review the elderly person's situation following the placement.

Elderly people in the sample were asked, 'Who decided on private residential care?'. Table 8.3 illustrated that thirty eight (19 per cent) of the decisions to enter private residential care were made by professionals alone, the majority of these (55 per cent) being decisions of a social worker. Social workers were, therefore, influential among professionals in this field in relation to decision-making.

Who were social workers making decisions for?
Professionals were involved in decision-making primarily in situations where the elderly person was confused (in 63 per cent of the cases where the social worker decided on residential care there was a decision taken on behalf of a confused person; 37 per cent where the person was not confused). Statements of social workers reflected this. For example:

> I'll decide for people if I feel they need to be pushed or they are mentally incapable.

Professionals made decisions for other groups of elderly people who were vulnerable, for example, those who lived alone (68 per cent of professionals made the decision where people lived alone).

In respect of these 24 people above, social workers saw no boundary to their role and transferred or extended their skills from the local authority to private settings, considering the private sector as an extra resource:

> I'll place a client in the same way - I'll ring round, look for a vacancy and try and work out where the individual would fit in... Very often you can't do that in our homes, you've got to go for the first vacancy.

A small number of social workers (two from hospital settings) totally immersed themselves in the private sector operation and saw their role not only in building links but acting as consultants by putting in specialist help and supporting private sector staff. One even encouraged residents to move from local authority to private homes.

Some social workers who placed elderly people in private homes felt their responsibility extended to a formal four or six week review which not only considered the individual resident but was used by some of them to 'informally keep a check on the home itself' and 'to keep home owners on their toes'.

Analysis of role

Although the majority of home owners (74 per cent) said that social workers were one source of referral (Chapter Seven), social workers were marginally involved in the process of admission into private residential care for elderly people. Two-thirds of the residents entered care without social work assistance; either they did not request a social work service or the social worker did not wish to become involved.

The professional social work service provided to the minority varied enormously. Where social workers actively engaged their skills outside the realms of the public sector, they fulfilled a variety of roles - providing information, giving advice to relatives and potential residents, recommending various private homes, and assessing the suitability of individual people for particular residential settings, negotiating the placement and enabling the admission.

They also took on roles other than those traditionally seen in the public sector such as an inspectoral role and consultative role to private home owners and managers.

The variability in role and level of involvement (some took on a marginal or cautious role, others became fully involved in the private sector admission), however, meant that elderly people received an unequal service. Whether the elderly person was given a choice and a social work service or not depended very often on which social worker they were allocated and the social worker's perspective of their role in the private sector.

Social workers in one field team viewed the private sector as exploitative and felt they should not be instrumental in making the selection between resources leading to private profit. Not only were they opposed to private care, but they felt that colleagues in other teams failed to offer an available alternative to residential care by readily making use of the private sector.

Although agency statements illustrated a commitment to a community care initiative, the group of social workers described above believed that the lack of resources going into such community packages put the client at risk and reflected in reality the agency's low level of commitment. In this particular geographical area, the field work team had developed packages of care to keep elderly mentally infirm people at home with support both from formal and informal sources, and were able to support very confused clients at home for long periods of time.

In the same catchment area, a very different perspective was found among the hospital team who came into contact with the same elderly people who entered hospital when their support systems broke down and relatives could no longer cope. Hospital social workers saw the only realistic placement for severely confused elderly people in a long-term 'secure' setting. They believed 'time and place become meaningless and therefore choice was non-existent'. From the perspective of one social worker, the limits on home care for such clients were much narrower:

> In a significant number of cases of chronic brain failure, there is nothing to be gained from continuing home care, other than perhaps the sacrificing of many people's needs in the often mistaken belief that home care is the only care and that failure to realise that meaningful and timely residential care can be the positive solution of all to all.

The stance taken by the field social worker against using residential care while insisting that the liberty of the individual was paramount and thereby keeping elderly people at home, was seen as unrealistic.

When GPs referred elderly people on to the psycho-geriatric team for assessment, the carefully laid plan of care at home provided by the field social worker was often overridden by hospital social workers operating independently of their colleagues.

Psychiatric hospital social workers viewed the field social workers as taking another ideological stance against private care, whereas field social workers refused, as a team, to admit people to private residential care. Private care was used consistently by the hospital team on the basis of availability and often proximity of the home to the resident's former residence. They had also built up intensive links with particular homes.

The variability of role also emerged because of the lack of clarity in the nature of social work as a profession. Chapter Two highlighted the fact that the nature of social work and its objectives were unclear in the public sector; evidence from this chapter shows that they are even more unclear when social work operates in a different sector of care. The basic principles of social work, such as individuality and client self-determination, and values such as choice were not upheld, through the political motivations of social workers operating in relation to the private sector.

The role of other professionals in the process

Other professionals, from the health sector in particular, also played a marginal role in the admission of elderly people into private residential care. As Table 8.1 shows, only thirty one people (15 per cent) said that their GP, community psychiatric nurse or health visitor were significantly involved in their process of admission. Other research studies (Phillips and Vincent, 1985b) show that GPs were not directly involved but operated via others, particularly social workers. It was interesting and surprising that health professionals were not more actively involved in the process of admission, particularly as private care gave them a resource to which they had relatively direct access, unlike public sector homes where they had to go through bureaucratic hurdles which probably involved a long wait for a vacancy.

However, the influence wielded by the medical profession on an individual's decision was far wider than the figures suggest. GPs were only marginally involved in the practicalities of an admission, but they influenced potential residents' self-perception and relatives' assessment of the situation facing the elderly person.

As Chapter Five highlighted, 62 residents (31 per cent) were advised against living alone by their GP or hospital doctor. Twelve GPs advised elderly people to enter residential care, while another three went further and phoned particular homes with which they had contact. Additional pressure by the GP was often exerted on relatives to 'do something' about their elderly relative. One daughter commented:

> The GP told us we'd have to push social services to do anything. (Daughter of Mrs Gilbert, Underwood)

Hospital doctors were involved in a number of admissions of confused elderly people into particular homes. The process from hospital to one particular home (Willow House) involved a number of health professionals working together. In this example, a particular network became established for confused people. Their entry into the system through contact with community psychiatric nurses (CPN) or certain social workers channelled them through 'classic' routes i.e. from psychiatric hospital, returning home with CPN support, until a private home was found. In most of these admissions the CPNs bypassed the social work service.

Very few 'other' professionals outside health and social services agencies, were actively involved in admissions. In such instances, 'professionals' played specific roles. Two solicitors were engaged to find a suitable home; church ministers were involved in practical and emotional support during the move for two elderly people. Others, an occupational therapist and a health visitor were initially involved in rehabilitation and then latterly in helping the elderly person decide on a move. An Age Concern volunteer was involved in one case and a DHSS officer in another, both giving financial advice.

Fully independent consumer

An elderly person who wished to enter a private home could do so without involving anyone else in the process. Professionals and relatives did not hold a unique position in the process of negotiation and, unlike entry to public sector residential resources, there was no obligation to seek a social worker assessment.

Eleven per cent (22) of people going into private homes went through the process independently. Very few were, therefore, 'consumers' in the true sense of the word.

Did this group consist of particular people?

In order to manage the process, a certain amount of information about the range of provision and ability to negotiate entry was necessary. This was reflected in the kind of resident found to be entering 'under their own steam'. Physically, they were able-bodied (73 per cent were independent) and in a good state of mental health (86 per cent were never confused).

Reasons for admission

1. A central recurring reason for seeking entry tended to be the fear of facing the future alone. Fifteen of those specifying no other significant people in their process of admission lived alone and were pessimistic about their ability to cope alone in the future:

> No-one else was involved. It's OK if you've got children, you can live on your own as they come and see you, but it's different and difficult for single people. You just have to look after yourself. (Mrs Hawkins, Elizabeth House)

2. For three people an advertised vacancy in the home triggered their admission. In some instances they had placed their names on the waiting list several months or years prior admission, to waiting for a particular room in a certain home:

> We made the decision ourselves and looked round and put our name on the waiting list one year before. (Mr and Mrs Plymouth, Oaklands)

Three residents entered after a bereavement of their partner. Another two entered because of loneliness, and three after inadequate support which they felt over a long period of time.

3. Four elderly people entered directly following an accident. Although these people were physically independent, two said a background reason for admission was their physical deterioration. Someone like Mrs Taylor (The Copse) fitted this description:

> It was my own decision. I was so frightened of being alone after my heart attack, I looked at the list while still in hospital and negotiated it myself.

This group planned their admission and entered in a straightforward manner after the negotiations were completed. Evidence indicated that a number of people had time to 'shop around' various homes, talk to Citizens' Advice Bureau workers and social security officers regarding their financial arrangements. Seventeen of these people were admitted from their own homes.

In all these cases, the elderly person did not recognise the need for a social worker to help them. They knew the kind of setting in which they wished to live and were able to go through the process unaided.

This group of people were empowered by the private sector process of admission; they made decisions themselves and nearly half (41 per cent) entered homes they chose because they themselves liked the home. (18 per cent entered because of recommendation; 14 per cent because it was near relatives). These were all positive choices made by prospective residents. Only two people felt they had made the wrong selection and put this down to not taking the time to look around, just taking the first vacancy.

Such self-determination in time and place of entry was restricted in a local authority residential admission. Yet nineteen people described in this section may not have been eligible for local authority residential because they were physically fit, mentally alert, not viewed as 'problems' and did not face a situation in which they were finding it difficult to cope. In consultation with other professionals, alternative resources may have prevented their entry into private residential care.

The other factor to be considered here is that a number were not in search of care and attention but saw the residential home as providing alternative accommodation, or viewed the home as a hotel, enabling them to come and go as they pleased (only one kept a house outside).

> I just wanted alternative accommodation. I'm very healthy and independent so I searched myself and chose not to involve anyone. (Miss Pigeon, Gracelands)

> There were no influences whatsoever. I chose it like a holiday. (Mrs Gable, Eastcliffe)

This lady was very unhappy and, on reflection, felt she drifted into this situation unknowingly.

Self-determination applied to those who were physically able to search, mentally alert to negotiate the placement, wealthy enough to choose between a range of provision which they liked, and who were able to enter at their own convenience. These people were the fully 'independent' consumers in the process. Such consumers, although small in number, exercised their rights of choice and extended their personal freedom in the private sector, not constrained by professional and bureaucratic hurdles.

However, without 'others' involved individual responsibility increased and, with the lack of an alternative 'viewing point', two people felt they had made the 'wrong' choice.

Discussion: The relationship between key operators in the process of admission

The decision taken by elderly people to enter either public or private care was determined less by particular circumstances and events than by the key concepts of finance, social class, availability of a vacancy and influential 'others' (Chapters 5 and 6).

This chapter illustrated that elderly people themselves could be over-ridden by relatives, ignored by social workers, rejected by home owners and pressured by relatives and GPs. Of all the outside influences, relatives were powerful advocates and directors of the process, sometimes through their own choice, at the request or inability of the elderly person (particular if they were confused) or through the withdrawal of the social worker for professional or political reasons in the process of admission to private care.

Unlike admission to public sector homes, social workers were not the main operators. They could have transferred their traditional skills of assessment and judgements about need in relation to the individual's unique circumstances to the private sector, yet social workers were marginally involved. Their lack of involvement in this sector was either because 'other' significant operators did not want them involved or because the social workers themselves did not wish to become involved. Relatives saw social workers as gatekeepers to local authority provision and saw no role for them in the private sector. Where they were involved there was an inconsistency in service provided to people entering private care. The same elderly people could go to different social workers, operating under different criteria, based on their personal and professional values and experience and, as a result, receive a very different service.

Recent reports, such as Griffiths (DHSS, 1988) and Wagner (1988) highlighted in Chapter Two, want to increase the social worker's role in the private sector. The literature related to this assumes that social workers can readily transfer their skills from one sector to another. In light of the fact that social workers played such a marginal role in the process and that the majority of relatives and residents (and home owners) were happy and satisfied with their 'choice' (Chapter Six), *is there a role for the social worker in the process of admission to private residential care?*

Home owners' evidence

The majority of home owners did not acknowledge or attach significance to the social work role in the process of admission. Most owners (22) said their relationship with social workers was poor. The seventeen owners who specified their 'good' relationship were in contact with particular social workers, usually from specialist settings (hospital based or the social worker for visually handicapped people).

Apart from their role as initial referrers, home owners viewed social work involvement as unnecessary and often 'interfering'. Their professional assessments were sometimes referred to as 'dubious' and 'suspicious', and they saw the assessment of residents in private care used against them with social workers deterring people from the home because it was not suited to the needs of the elderly person. They saw a medical assessment demanding the skills of a GP but, as far as a social assessment was concerned, they felt capable to coming to a conclusion themselves with the help of relatives: there was no necessary role for a social worker. Some home owners said social workers only appeared when they were desperate, as those from the Risings and Rosehill comment:

> The social worker only appears when there's a crisis and when the family want to dump their elderly relative in a home.
>
> We have as little contact as possible with them. They are never there when you want them and then they only interfere.

The traditional role of the social worker was redundant in the private sector as far as home owners were concerned. No home owner involved a social worker in their assessment stage as a routine matter of procedure.

Health service professionals in relation to social workers played a greater role in the eyes of the home owners, with nine homes (23 per cent) always calling for a formal medical report. The inclusion of GPs and exclusion of social workers reflected the high status and regard felt by home owners for the medical profession, particularly among those owners coming from a nursing background.

A closer look at the local authority's current relationship with the private sector suggested, therefore, that there were difficulties, particularly in terms of 'providing an adequate political and coherent professional response' (Willcocks, 1987, p.7).

As shown, on a political level the ideological commitments of some social workers did not fit easily with the development of pluralist welfare. Social workers, therefore, before assessing the need for private residential care will have to address their own value systems and political beliefs as well as their perceptions of private sector homes and their owners. If the client is to have confidence in social workers and to receive a fair and objective professional assessment, then some social workers must re-examine their views that all private sector homes are exploitive. Others placed a preference on a private resource. Variability in the levels of commitment and involvement need to be examined before the traditional skills of assessment become the task of the social worker in the private sector. Otherwise, the relationship between the two sectors will be a forced one with the social worker acting in an uncomfortable position as buffer or barrier between the two. Although the agency may be working towards a more positive approach, the service the client receives may not be positive.

It was not only the political motivations of social workers that distorted their role in the private sector: more fundamental principles of social welfare were at stake. The need for residential care was examined to gain entry into the public sector; criteria for admission into private care, however, was dictated by the market place, need was taken as the person's ability to pay. The social worker's role as assessor therefore was distorted because they were assessing the potential resident's need in relation to community care in the public sector whereas a different model of assessment operated in private care, with felt need not being evaluated against community alternatives but ability to pay.

Even within the private sector itself, different philosophies of care operated, depending on the background of the home owner and the dependency characteristics of the residents. In other words, there was no agreed procedure for admission or for assessing need in the private sector.

Evidence from the Suffolk study found that assessment remained in the hands of one person, the home owner, with very few homes engaged in employing an outside professional opinion.

The traditional role of the social worker was distorted by these factors in the private sector. If the social worker's role is to be increased in this sector as suggested, for example, by Wagner (1988) and Firth (DHSS, 1987) then there are several points to consider in relation to social work skills.

Extra skills/knowledge required of social workers in the private sector

1. The social worker will be obliged to be knowledgeable about the whole spectrum of different resources private homes can offer. They will need to expand their knowledge which will mean extending involvement with the private sector. This is necessary because the criteria for admission will be based on local authority experience and will be different from those operated in the private sector. This demands a knowledge of the assessment and admission process of other key operators and particularly the home owner. However, the research does show that to some extent some social workers are already doing this. Many already have a good rapport working for the benefit of their clients.

2. There is a need for careful matching of client need and resource. If the social worker is assessing the 'best' option for the client, this should include 'matching the right person to the right home' (BASW, 1984, p.9). Variability of provision will make the task of careful matching complex, particularly with the existence of dually registered homes falling into both residential and nursing home criteria. Social workers will not only need to be knowledgeable about such provision, but will be required to assess between different levels of care, between those in need of residential care and those needing nursing care. As Abrams (1978) describes, social workers will need to extend their role and become para-medical workers.

3. To do a 'good' job for the client places a duty on social workers not only to cover all aspects of assessment in depth but to guide the elderly person through entry into care. This will not only increase costs to both sectors but will imply huge resource implications for the public sector in particular. A direct consequence of assessing someone suitable for care, deems them eligible for public care also. Alongside this, if clients are not in need of residential care in the light of community resources, then such resources must be acceptable and accessible to the client. Further to this, the circumstances and needs of clients change over time; the social worker must be equipped to monitor these changes and make sure they offer effective alternatives to residential care in the community which increases the role of the social worker and costs to the agency.

4. One of the readings of the Griffiths Report (DHSS, 1988) is to make a social work service available to all persons thinking about residential care. Even if this only applied to those seeking state finance, the implications are enormous. The Suffolk study revealed that only 48 per cent of those residents receiving DHSS funding received help from social workers. To increase the service to cover all such applicants would be a sizeable increase with vast resource implications.

Finally, the consequences of increased professional power via assessment are at the sacrifice of client choice, particularly for those not in any professionally defined need for residential care. Thirty seven per cent of those receiving DHSS support in the Suffolk study felt there was no other effective alternative other than entering a private home. A minority of such people entered for peace of mind and security reasons, viewing a private home as an alternative housing option rather than a care facility; others came to relieve their fear of future frailty, particularly if they lived alone. For those people, increasing professional power would mean an existence of 'enforced independence' in the community.

This chapter highlights that the traditional role of social workers in the process of admission into local authority homes (see Chapter Two) was taken by relatives in the admission to private residential homes. The majority of residents, relatives and home owners saw no necessity to involve social workers and the fact that a group of elderly people, although small in number, entered residential care independently of others, demonstrated this. One area in which all parties felt social workers to be legitimate was in relation to the admission of confused elderly people. Otherwise their role was marginal and inconsistent.

At present, the private sector, however, cannot stand alone. With the injection of public money, it has to be publicly accountable and therefore have local authority involvement. Although the local authority is statutorily bound to work with the private sector in terms of registration, regulation and inspection, the basis for social workers to become involved is not as clear cut, although under the National Assistance Act 1948, local authorities have a duty to provide accommodation for those elderly people in need and the private sector can be used.

The skills thought necessary by home owners to work alongside the private sector were those not commonly thought of as social work practitioner skills; for instance, planning experience, managing a business, or skills in inter-agency work. The skills social workers possessed, particularly in professionally assessing the need for residential care, were redundant in the private sector.

The expectation, therefore, that social workers will automatically play a larger role in the private sector by transferring their traditional skills of assessment, needs to be closely examined. This study revealed that their role was distorted in the private sector, not only because they operated in two models of care which conflicted, but their personal, professional and political preferences, along with their confusion over agency policy, resulted in an unequal and inconsistent service to elderly people. Such conflicts were reflected by 'others' ignoring the professionals and organising their future direction of care in the private market themselves or with the help of relatives.

When assessment of those seeking public funding becomes the task of the social worker, then there is a need to clarify involvement and objectives of assessment in order to allow elderly people a fair service. Otherwise, separate systems will emerge: one for the 'deserving rich' - those who can determine their own entry into care, and another for the 'deserving poor' - those entering the system after multiple assessment, involving bureaucratic hurdles dictated by both the market (price) and by professional judgements (social planning mechanisms).

9 The process of admission into private residential care

In this chapter an attempt will be made to draw together the main findings of the study and to discuss their implications for policy and practice in the private sector of residential care for elderly people. It will be argued that there are fewer differences than might have been expected between the populations of residents in the public and private sectors, but that the presence of and role played by social workers appears to be a critical factor.

In the course of presenting the argument, generalisations will be made which, it is believed, accurately reflect the picture that has emerged during the empirical phases of the study. There are, of course, always exceptions, but a sufficiently clear perspective can be obtained to allow us to draw conclusions about the private sector and how its residents gain admission.

1. Who enters private residential care?

A number of wide-ranging analyses were conducted in an attempt to identify the differences between the residents of private care and those living in local authority homes. From a number of key variables, statistically significant differences emerged only in respect of mental state, social class and home ownership: Public sector residents were more likely to be confused (though not in vast proportions); they tended to come from a lower social class, and they generally lived in rented accommodation.

In respect of age, sex, marital status and physical dependency, there were no differences between the sectors, and this finding reflected the important fact that the residents of private homes were in most ways typical of the 'old elderly' British population as a whole. Indeed, it might be asserted that the residents of private residential care were not in any obvious way 'unusual': they represented a cross-section of 'old elderly' people, many of whom sooner or later feel the need for a degree of residential care.

Residential homes in the private sector provided a service for 'typical' older members of society - mainly widowed females over the age of 75 years. Other groups, married or single men or women, or those under the age of 75, were not excluded, but they were present in homes only in smaller proportions.

Although private residential care is now potentially available, through income maintenance schemes, to all 'older elderly' people, a clear majority in the Suffolk sample were not dependent on DHSS funding. It can therefore be said that, at the present time, although there is no deliberate exclusion of poorer elderly people from private homes, the sector nevertheless caters principally for more wealthy elderly people not reliant on state funding.

Not only were these elderly people 'typical' in terms of their basic profile but they entered a home through circumstances usually experienced by all those who enter residential care i.e. a decline in health and breakdown of support. Although on a dependency scale, the majority of residents were physically independent (ie they could wash, dress and walk unaided) and were not mentally confused; 89 per cent had a background of some degree of physical or mental frailty, which required support in a number of ways from family and from professional care services, such as health visitors or social workers. A breakdown in their family support system often meant that they were unable to remain independent in the community.

The move into private residential care, therefore, was not experienced by a select group of elderly people who made a conscious decision to enter care shortly after retirement, but by a whole range of older members of society as a reaction to the deteriorating circumstances in which they found themselves.

2. What is the nature of private residential care?

Elderly people entered a homely, caring environment, described by one home owner as a 'homely hotel with care'.

The various kinds of provision and styles of operation that home owners offered corresponded with the expectations of their consumers. Everyone's image of old age could be accommodated by such variety of provision, whether it be a quiet retreat at a country cottage, a small home overlooking the sea or an ordinary house in suburbia.

Despite the heterogeneity of residential provision in this sector in terms of location, external appearance and operational style, the majority of the thirty nine homes attempted to recreate 'the caring family'. This was most apparent in those homes run jointly by husband and wife, sometimes employing a network of their family to help carry out different tasks required in the business.

Alongside the family model of care, home owners were eager to present a 'professional' image which was most apparent in their emphasis on a medical orientation in the style of care they displayed. Many home owners took the view that a nursing qualification enhanced their credibility in the eyes of relatives, who mostly approached home owners because of their own inability to continue in a caring and supportive practical role to their frail parent. It was also important to relatives that their elderly parent 'enjoyed' the security offered by qualified staff being available twenty-four hours a day. Relatives were less concerned with the home owners attempts at maximising the independence of residents or allowing the elderly person to take risks and were more interested in or anxious about the 'security' offered in suitable accommodation with a family orientated atmosphere.

Few homes operated purely along medical lines: the majority scored favourably in terms of the extent to which they afforded a degree of independence to residents alongside the provision of privacy, care and homeliness. Such aspects which family living ideally provides supported the idea that care in a homely environment was a main feature of private residential care. There was very little evidence found in this study to support the idea of the private sector 'exploiting' vulnerable people for profit by accommodating them in inappropriate, spartan or uncaring conditions.

Although the majority of home owners said that their initiative in setting up a home was not led primarily by the profit motive, they were, on the other hand not altruistic. In running a business they needed to balance the books and achieving this objective was one of the biggest initial headaches mentioned by many proprietors, particularly if structural alterations and refurbishing were necessary. In a number of cases the husband worked outside the home in his own business in order to supplement their income. For other home owners who welcomed the opportunity to work together, diversifying outside the residential care business was less attractive; they consequently found other ways to make ends meet, for example by setting fees higher than the DHSS limits and restricting entry to those who were able to meet the fees themselves rather than relying on DHSS support.

The majority of home owners, however, demonstrated that professional standards of care can be provided within a profitable business framework.

The family image of private residential care, with home owners and their families providing a personal service within a domestic and 'secure' atmosphere, was an attractive feature to elderly people and their families. That image was marketed profitably by home owners.

3. Were residents satisfied with private residential care?

The majority of residents and their relatives were happy with the package of residential care on offer. The different types and styles of provision available corresponded with consumer expectations. Physical features, both internal and external, were seen as being very important: the external appearance and location of the home were important for attracting potential customers, and consumer satisfaction was influenced by room size and the quality of the furnishings. Privacy in the form of single room accommodation was paramount for a majority of respondents. Less tangible features around the elements of staff care and services such as good food also ranked high in satisfaction scores. The caring and coping skills of home owners and their staff were frequently mentioned by families who had struggled to cope in difficult and 'impossible' situations for a number of years. Some professionals, too, praised staff for their ability to manage often the most difficult residents and in two specialist homes for their skills in relation to people with mental infirmity. Relatives in particular commented not only on how well residents were cared for but also on the 'personable' and 'approachable' nature of staff members.

Where there were expressions of dissatisfaction they focused both on the poor quality of care provided and on the inferior physical standards in the home.

In general, the components of private residential care were attractive and consumers were satisfied with the facilities on offer. Consequently, there was very little emphasis placed on widespread advertising with the market led by demand from elderly people and their relatives.

4. The role of relatives

The majority of elderly people had relatives who supported and sustained them in the community and when unable to continue this function, helped them find a suitable residential home.

The influence of relatives prior to admission was considerable. Informal family networks, rather than professional sources were important in keeping elderly people in the community. The evidence suggested that it was very often a breakdown in the family's ability to sustain their caring relationship in some very vulnerable situations that initiated the move into private residential care. In such cases, the relative decided that they could no longer cope with the care demands of their elderly mother or father or aunt, particularly if they were confused. In most cases this was not in conflict with the wishes of elderly people who did not want to become a burden on their carer, particularly by moving to live with them.

Relatives were also influential in choosing the home and negotiating with the home owner. The presence of a son or daughter often meant an absence of a professional as relatives took it upon themselves to find a suitable private home and did not see the need to involve a social worker. They saw it as their responsibility in the first instance to seek an appropriate setting. Relatives were more likely to consider a private sector home than a public sector one for a number of reasons. Private residential care provided a flexible service to relatives. Unlike entry to public sector provision there was no necessity to go through a bureaucratic process. There was also no professional assessment of the elderly person's need for residential care or of the relative's need for relief.

The absence of a professional also meant that relatives turned to the sector where they could negotiate directly with a number of home owners, who probably would provide the day to day support for their elderly parent. They could negotiate directly the timing of entry to suit them and they could visit a number of homes and gain first hand experience of the market, rather than be led to one home by a professional decision. Relatives also believed that they had more chance of getting their elderly mother into a private home than a public sector one and, therefore, naturally turned to this sector first. In seeking a home, relatives saw themselves taking on the traditional role of a social worker.

5. The role of the social worker

The one major difference between public and private sector residents lay in the extent to which social workers were involved in the process of admission. The majority of elderly people did not engage a social worker to help them enter a private home. Social workers were not seen in a unique role as gatekeepers to private sector provision, information brokers or advocates in the process of admission. Relatives also did not see the need to employ them to find a suitable home. They were seen purely as gatekeepers to local authority resources and when there were no vacancies in local authority care (or relatives thought there would not be a vacancy) they did not see the social worker in any further role, apart from giving them a list of registered private homes in the county. They were seen as rationing agents, partly defined through their agency function in relation to local authority care. Relatives and their parents saw social workers providing access to a residential service and when this could not be obtained they saw their role as redundant.

Some social workers confirmed this perception. When they could not provide an appropriate placement in the public sector, as agents of that sector, they did not see their role extending into the private sector. They clearly saw it as the function of the family to negotiate between elderly people and the home owner and in some cases the social worker went to great lengths to find a family to act on behalf of the 'client'. Social workers in this group were reluctant to become involved in the 'private relationship' that existed between families and home owners.

Some elderly people entered private residential care through marginal contact with a social worker. In some instances, families who had initial contact with social workers chose to ignore them or bypassed them by going through other professional channels. This was particularly evident in cases involving confused people who were in danger of floating around the care system waiting for a public sector vacancy. Medical networks operating together with particular private homes enabled health professionals to acquire suitable vacancies without involving social workers.

Other elderly people received a marginal service from professionals because social workers acting as public sector agents were confused as to how far they could assist the elderly person to enter a private home. Without clear practical agency guidelines, social workers were left to use their personal and professional discretion as to whether they enabled elderly people and their families to pursue a private sector placement. In some cases, their political preferences were expressed; being opposed to private care, they withdrew and left elderly people and their families to pursue a course into private residential care.

In a minority of instances, social workers became actively involved and guided elderly people through a bureaucratic process similar to the process of admission into local authority residents care - they assessed the elderly person's need for care and entered into negotiation with home owners to find a suitable placement. Some social workers only took on this role when there was no family to help the elderly person.

Some social workers saw this relationship with the private sector as 'forced' and 'necessary' because of the lack of public sector vacancies and were cautious in their approach. Other social workers expressed a personal and political preference for the private sector and enthusiastically and comfortably worked alongside the family in the process of admission. Some believed that private residential care offered a better and more flexible deal to elderly people and their relatives, and a small number of such social workers, particularly among those who were hospital based, saw themselves assisting home owners as gatekeepers to private sector provision. The majority of hospital social workers held favourable views of the private sector, building up and tapping their networks in that sector whenever necessary.

Very few elderly people entered private residential care entirely as 'independent' agents without help from relatives or professional carers in the process of admission. Few 'shopped around' and chose what they saw as the most suitable provision.

Elderly people, their relatives and social workers themselves, did not consider a social work service vital in the process of admission to a private residential home. The traditional role of a social worker in facilitating admission could be undertaken by relatives.

6. How do potential residents choose between homes?

(i) Choice within the private sector

In selecting a home, consumers in the free market expressed preferences for small homes offering privacy and care, with sufficient flexibility to accommodate their individual tastes. However, they were often constrained in their choice by the home owner's admissions criteria which related to physical and mental state as well as to the individual's ability to pay. Those prospective residents who were confused or supported financially by the state were more likely than any other group of people to lack choice in the private sector: in Suffolk they had free access to twenty five out of the thirty-nine homes studied. Applicants dependent on DHSS funding were excluded from twenty of the thirty nine homes studied. Despite the impression of variety in private sector provision, a free choice of home was not available, therefore, to all potential residents and their relatives.

The process of admission was not straightforward. Even if the would-be resident passed the admissions criteria operating in a particular home, there might simply not be a vacancy there at the appropriate time; the result would be that they simply sought the next nearest available and appropriate vacancy.

(ii) Choice within the public sector

In comparison with the private sector the public sector was never designed to give residents freedom of choice between homes. Client choice played only a small part in the bureaucratic decision making process with the eventual outcome usually constrained by geographical boundaries and professional assessment.

The evidence confirmed that few public sector residents had been given a choice between two or more public sector homes.

(iii) Choice between the public and the private sector

Although it is recognised that doctors, relatives and social workers exercise some influence over the choice of a home, the related surveys of residents in public and private sectors revealed a larger-than-expected number who appeared to have had no strong preference for one or the other. This can be shown diagrammatically:

DIAGRAM 9.1
THE PERCENTAGES OF RESIDENTS WHO EXERCISE A PREFERENCE FOR PRIVATE OR PUBLIC SECTOR CARE

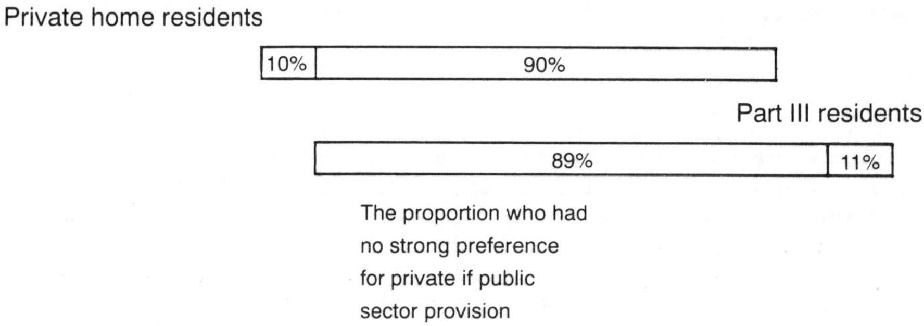

Only a minority of elderly people expressed a preference for one sector or the other. Where there was a conscious decision made to enter private care rather than public sector care it was based on the perception of local authority provision as lacking privacy, being shabby or housing 'riff-raff'. Others choose private sector provision because the wait for a bed in a local authority home appeared long and the bureaucratic process could not guarantee to result in a vacancy in a particular home of their choice.

Only a small minority held political beliefs against privatization and preferred to enter public sector provision for that reason. The majority of public sector residents believed they were excluded from the private sector because of their lack of finance. Where they were able to apply for state funding, the lack of appropriate private home vacancies restricted them.

Why did the 90 per cent of residents who were not committed to one sector or the other end up in a particular sector of care? Few residents were strongly opposed to one sector: private sector residents, in other words, would have entered a local authority home if they had known that suitable vacancies existed.

The majority of residents were forced by deteriorating circumstances to look at the variety of residential provision. Their lack of confidence in community supports made them unable to remain independent at home. The majority also did not want to become a burden on their relatives and as an alternative to living with them, they pursued a place in a residential home. Wealthier sections of the elderly population did not have greater choice between staying put and going into a home. Very few people bought private domiciliary care, which indicated that what wealth they had was tied up in their property and, therefore, they could only use it by going into residential care: it was not an available asset for use while resident in the community.

Although few people expressed a preference, they did not enter the private sector purely by chance: elderly people were steered by the actions of their relatives to look first to the private sector. The final decision, therefore, to enter a private home often involved a compromise between key operators in the process. In other words, it was not a decision taken primarily by elderly people but by their relatives.

The choice of home within the private sector was surprisingly restricted. Despite the variety of provision, which, in theory, provided some real alternatives, only a minority could exercise choice: the majority were constrained by the home owner's restrictive practices, by their own geographical preference, their financial standing and by the availability of a suitable place at the crucial time.

In reality there was little evidence of 'shopping around' after placement. Once in a home, a resident was more likely to stay there even if dissatisfied. Six per cent of residents in the private sector had moved within the private sector in the previous year, many because their relatives were unhappy with the conditions they were in; ten per cent moved from one public sector home to another.

No evidence was found of residents who moved from a private sector to a public sector home, or vice versa. The movement was therefore, within and not between sectors. No home owners rejected residents in large numbers once they were admitted. In addition, it was found that in the majority of homes (64 per cent), all of the residents interviewed were happy and satisfied.

Implications for social work practice in the process of admission to private residential care

The key distinction between the private and public sector was the presence and role played by key negotiators and operators in the process. The presence of a close relative in the admission process, which often meant the lack of a professional, was a determining factor in entry to the private sector.

In the public sector the process of admission was managed and organised by a social worker with the ultimate choice of home decided following professional assessment. The preferences of elderly people, and particularly of their relatives, were marginal to the process. The lack of a similar professional assessment in private sector admissions has worried those who feel that elderly people enter private residential care unnecessarily. Some (*The Griffiths Report*, DHSS, 1988; BASW quoted in Morris, 1986) go further than this by saying that social workers should be involved in such assessments if private residential care is to be part of the arena of welfare as a whole. Those people not in a professionally defined 'need' of residential care are seen to be wasting scarce resources better allocated to those genuinely in need of a residential place.

Wagner, in *A Positive Choice* (1988), argues that all residential care packages should include a social work service. This she defines as:

1. Practical advice and help in coping with day to day problems and counselling when needed (p.21).

2. Specialised programmes of care, assessment, treatment and rehabilitation.

3. Social workers acting as family agents, giving information and providing help with decision making in relation to the admission process.

Should a social worker be involved in private sector admissions?

From the evidence presented in this study, it could be argued that for elderly people with relatives who could assist them in the process of admission there was no need for a social worker to be involved. Relatives were able to act as information brokers, decision makers and negotiators in the entry to private residential care. Social workers were primarily seen as decision makers for public sector residential care alone or for those elderly people without relatives, or where relatives were unable or unwilling to assist them.

At the extreme it could be argued that social workers should not be involved at all in the private sector admission process, firstly because of the lack of clear agency function in the private sector, and secondly, as a result of this, because of the inconsistent service elderly people received from social workers.

It could also be argued that the social worker has no clear role through the lack of agency function and objectives. Taft (1944) comments:

> When there is no supporting medium, such as the social agency supplies, no application process through which the applicant may test relation to agency and to the service he apparently seeks, there is, in my opinion, no place for the social worker. He himself may become the service, as the therapist does, but he no longer operates his own unique profession. (p.265)

Private sector growth has challenged and focused attention on the relationships between the individual's autonomy and agency objectives.

It could also be argued that the presence of a social worker in the process of admission was inappropriate because without any agency guidelines, social workers acted autonomously and provided an inconsistent service to elderly people. The study showed that social workers were confused about their agency's line with regard to operating in the private arena. Of those who thought there was a particular strategy outlined by the agency, half thought they could only give a list and not recommend particular homes, while the other half thought the policy was to fully promote both sectors. Despite such confusion, the majority of social workers overruled this and 'did their own thing', either based on their ideological stance or on what they saw as best for the client; for example, giving a list to a confused client was seen as pointless unless the vetting and negotiation of admission was undertaken by the social worker.

Social workers demonstrated autonomy in relation to three areas which Howe (1979) defines as:

1. Their definition of the task (ie whether there was a need to counsel people with regard to other options or to promote the process of admission into private residential care or whether there was any task to be performed).

2. Their definition of the client. (Some social workers exerted their personal discretion to work with those clients who they saw needed residential care and wanted private care and had the ability to pay. Other social workers rejected anyone wishing to enter private care regardless of need).

3. A definition of their relationship with the client (and private sector). Some social workers saw their role as inconsistent with their individual values and saw no moral commitment to engage in a relationship with the elderly person. Others viewed it as a 'relationship of necessity' while another group participated in a relationship with the client taking them through the process of admission.

Although the nature of social work calls for the social worker to exercise a degree of personal autonomy in assessment and decision making and, therefore, there cannot be any hard standard criteria, the extent of social worker autonomy in the private sector was inappropriate because of the implications of their actions.

Whether they withdrew their involvement or fully participated in the process of admission, because they favoured one system over the other, they denied elderly people access to alternative choices. Full scale liaison, for instance, patronising and operating fully within the private sector to the exclusion of the public sector, undermined the raison d'etre of social work itself and in this way was inappropriate. Whether elderly people were afforded choice or not depended on the particular social worker to whom they were allocated, and as a result, social workers promoted a very unfair and unequal service.

A balance needs to be struck, therefore, as to the appropriate role and level of involvement in this sector with the social worker helping those genuinely in 'need'. This could include those elderly people without relatives to help them through the process.

Elderly people without relatives and those who are socially isolated should have access to a social work service as outlined by Wagner (1988). Social workers, as agents of welfare should be involved in building up a body of knowledge about all forms of welfare, including the private sector, and act as information brokers for those elderly people without family to support them. Whether elderly people have financial resources or not, the social worker can play a legitimate role, not only in defining need but also by matching that particular need to suitable provision. They can also fulfil traditional roles in terms of monitoring and coordinating packages of care (see Chapter One).

There is no reason why social workers acting as family agents should not liaise with the private sector in this way. However, the relationship between home owners and social workers needs to be addressed if professional social workers are to take an active part in assessment and admission on behalf of the family otherwise elderly people will receive a different service depending on the social worker allocated.

The local authority will have to clearly outline its function in the private sector and home owners will have to accept a certain amount of professional intrusion in their relationship with residents.

The reports of Wagner (1988), Firth (DHSS, 1987) and Griffiths (DHSS, 1988) see social workers as public sector agents becoming more intrusive in the private sector. This study, however, would advocate a diminutive role for social workers where elderly people have relatives to assist them in the process of admission (particularly if the conclusion of Gibbs and Bradshaw, 1988, is correct: that is, the majority of people in private voluntary homes for the elderly were in need of residential care at the time of admission). Social workers, however, should be available to those without family to help them with admission. If needs assessment of all applicants for income support becomes a reality then the social worker should withdraw after 'need for care' has been assessed, leaving the relative (where possible) to carry through the process of admission.

This conclusion is not only based on evidence of a lack of clear agency function for social workers in the private sector, but on evidence presented by relatives and elderly people on their perceptions of the social worker's role in the private residential care system.

All significant parties in the process of admission (elderly people, their relatives and home owners) saw social workers primarily as rationing agents, allocating scarce beds to those most in need in the public sector. They did not see their role extending into the private sector in terms of finding the most suitable provision on behalf of elderly people but saw social workers blocking choice and depriving elderly people of private homes irrespective of need. Customers of the private sector recognised that social workers were primarily rationing provision even in this sector and, as a result, did not apply for a social work service but preferred to operate 'independently'. The relative did not see the social worker in a helpful guiding role.

Conclusion

Admission into private residential care was not achieved through the exercise of free market choice. Neither was it dependent upon bureaucratic processes. The majority of elderly people were forced by deteriorating home circumstances to seek residential care. Their relatives directed them to the private sector believing they had more chance of entering a residential home in this sector than in the public sector. Their eventual destination at a particular private home was decided by the availability of a place at the crucial time within a certain geographical area. Social workers took a back seat to relatives in this process.

There was no evidence to suggest that elderly people were unhappy about this process. The majority of elderly people voiced their satisfaction with the care they received within the privacy and comfort of their own room.

Postscript

The social work role in the 1990s

One of the central questions facing Social Services Departments in the 1990's is whether there is a role for social work with older people and if so, who should be providing it and what it should look like? This section considers these issues by looking at the Community Care Act 1990 and its consequences for Social Work and Social Workers with older people.

There has been little challenge to the social work role in relation to older people since the restructuring of social services following Seebohm. With the reorganisation, there existed an expectation that the profile of work with older people would be raised and the professionalism it required would be acknowledged. Research in the late 1970's and early 1980's shows how false this hope was with social work with older people being the task delegated to social work assistants. Anyone working in the arena of eldercare was seen to be committing professional suicide. Social workers with older people did not view themselves as change agents in a therapeutic sense. To the outside world social work with older people has been about arranging 'packages of care' and anyone could be forgiven for thinking that few professional skills were required to do the job.

The recent legislation accepts this view and as a result presents a direct challenge to the social work role vis a vis older people. The Community Care Act questions the very value base of social work itself and focuses attention on why and what special skills, knowledge and values are required to work in this area of welfare delivery. The independent and informal sectors are seen to be equally capable.

The access families need to good quality social work support in caring for older people has been ignored. It has only reemerged in the impending panic approaching the labour market with a potential lack of entrants into the workforce. Traditional female carers, married women in their 40's and 50's are being enticed back into the job market. Many such women are also caring for elderly people in the community. If these carers are to seriously re-enter the labour force then support to them is vital.

The new Act sees such support provided by the private and voluntary sectors.

Care management

Care management is inextricably bound to the ideological belief in the mixed economy of welfare. The components it espouses are related to promoting the development of an alternative sector of welfare. It has been argued by its critics (Jack, 1991) that care management is not a tool for enabling elderly people to exercise choice in the welfare market but for the erosion of social work with older people and the destruction of Local Authority state workers, who are seen as responsible for fostering a so called 'dependency culture' while undermining family values and responsibilities.

The rationale for the introduction of care management is based on the critique of SSD's by the Audit Commission whose main criticisms are that needs and services are not matched; there is a fragmentation of services and a lack of coordination at local level (Audit Commission, 1986). Such can be remedied through care management and SSD's are attracted to the concept on a number of fronts. It provides a new approach to home care through - targeting those in need

- providing smaller caseloads
- decentralised budgets
- closer health links
- and systematic recording

In other words, it is seen as a means of more effective and efficient organisation. However, the initial enthusiasm for care management is beginning to subside as further investigation finds it lacking a practice model in social work. It is much better suited as a tool for management. In terms of cost effectiveness it can work as Davies (Challis & Davies 1986) has shown, Griffiths (1988 p.vii) even dismisses the importance of the social work component:

> The role of the public sector is essentially to ensure that care is provided. How it is provided is an important, but secondary consideration...

In other words, the way in which care is delivered is not of primary importance; it does not necessarily require professional carers. Government guidance on care management is also interesting for what it omits as well as what it includes. It has little room for good social work practice to meet the needs of older people.

On an administrative level there is little suggestion that care management will provide smaller caseloads. Although there will be a concentration on a small number of high risk clients there will be a much larger number of clients requiring monitoring. Clients will get a less direct service but this does not necessarily mean a reduced caseload for social workers.

In this sense care management doesn't necessarily achieve its objective. In order to do so, SSD's must adopt systematic recording and recognise the need for better information technology which means resources need to be allocated to training. Social work as a profession has been slow to take on board the use of such technology in any significant way.

Although claimed as efficient, care management leads to a large increase in bureaucratic procedure. Assessment forms used in many areas are long and time consuming and allow little flexibility. The implication is that anyone can use them yet the 'hidden' agendas behind many referrals to social work departments require professional skills of assessment. Care management in this sense suits the needs of the organisation rather than the individual for whom it was designed.

Care management doesn't promote better practice in relation to direct work with clients. 'Caring for People' introduces the notion of a purchaser/provider split in the organisation in order to fulfil various policy objectives such as securing clear specifications of the services to be provided and the costs. The split suggests that the needs of older people can be easily disentangled and desegregated, with the purchaser concentrating on the assessment side of the social work function and the provider being seen as separate (and in the independent sector). Ongoing support and review in the long term is not seen as integral to both functions. For older people in residential care, where there is little or no family contact or involvement then it is important for the officer in charge to carry out both functions of review and provision as well as liaising with the social worker. The Act recognises the difficulty in separating these functions.

> advice/ongoing support role of social workers may suffer if purchaser activities of arranging services from third parties come to dominate. (DoH, 1991, p.25).

It becomes increasingly difficult to separate out the counselling from the care management role. Casework under the care management function will be seen in the provider function, yet casework is an important part of assessment which in the new Act has gone unrecognised. The quality of the relationship between the social worker and the client will also suffer if there is no continuity of support.

Assessment will also need to be multi-disciplinary, an area in which social workers are not on the whole skilled; they will also, because of this, need to command resources from other sectors or at least be knowledgeable about them. The White paper guidance, in answer to this, suggests that such multi-disciplinary elements of assessment can be sub-contracted (DoH, 1991 p.34) but this places the client and social worker further away in terms of direct contact.

Splitting the functions of social workers along purchaser/provider lines and sub-contracting elements of assessment will also be confusing for clients and their families. In this sense it mystifies the purpose and nature of social workers and the role of the social worker as care manager.

Social work with older people is seen in the new Act as purely a service provision task. Negotiating help is seen as a practical matter with any professional able to carry out an assessment and put together a package of care.

There has been little consideration of the unique holistic skills needed and adopted by social workers in carrying out assessment, which should take place between services and sectors and not narrowly within a service, which has been a frequent criticism of similar care professionals (Fisher, 1991, p15). The Act doesn't specify that social work skills are necessary in this area of assessment (DoH, 1990 3.34). The danger is therefore that the assessment of needs will be, to a greater extent than at present, service led.

The essential knowledge that social workers have regarding older people is also ignored as a component of case management. Will other personnel be equipped and trained (as ASW's for example) to assess a person requiring immediate treatment?

Social work values are also eroded. Will case management allow for self determination as a guiding principle or will clients be 'managed'? Will choice take a primary position if in conflict with cost-effectiveness? Fisher (1991) argues that case management on this basis doesn't enhance clients rights.

To avoid the destruction of social workers with older people then case management should be underpinned with social work values rather than economic principles. The Government want to promote an economic consciousness underlying the case management function yet there is little if any discussion of where social work fits in.

Case management is being introduced as a new tool yet the elements are little different from the ingredients of social work as it stands at present. Good social work practice starts with professional assessment on the basis of need; it also involves accessing resources and networking. The tone of the new act however, places emphasis on the need to change one's attitude and way of working. The legislation lays emphasis on new areas of accountability and undermines social work values while de-professionalising social work and hence marginalising social work as a core ingredient in working with older people.

Case management contains little that is new in social work practice. The jargon suggests otherwise, which is confusing for clients and social workers. The use of words such as customer and service user in itself has created an illusion of choice and empowerment which cannot be supported in relation to older people in practice, partly because there simply isn't a wide variety of provision to choose between.

The new elements for social workers taking on a case management role will be:-

1. Holding a budget
2. Working with and promoting external provision of resources

1. The 3e's of economy, efficiency and effectiveness have dominated the direction of SSD's over the last 10 years. The Audit Commission was concerned with these issues and was highly critical of social workers in this vein. The White paper specifies that LA's should find the most cost effective care choice from the private and voluntary sectors. This however appears a

Inability of family to continue caring

Problems associated with an informal carer provided another reason for admission (Tables 5.7 and 5.8). Lack of family support networks, either through the family's unwillingness or, to a greater extent, their inability to continue in a caring role, reinforced the vulnerability of those elderly people who suffered poor health or a deterioration in their mental state.

Forty two elderly people (21 per cent) came into private residential care directly as a result of the family's inability to support them at home; and 36 (18 per cent) of the residents who came into residential care for a variety of other reasons, had relatives who found it difficult to cope with the situation of caring for an elderly mother or aunt.

Families had particular difficulty in caring for people with poor physical health or where confused. Of those families with a confused elderly relative, 27 (65 per cent of the 42 families unable to continue caring) felt inadequately supported by formal and informal services. It was in such a situation of helplessness that a great deal of family support broke down and the point at which residential care was seen as the only solution.

Other elderly people were placed in a vulnerable position by a reversal of role with their immediate carer. The carer, whether it was wife, husband or daughter, often became ill and unable to continue in their supporting role which sometimes resulted in their admission to hospital.

Mr and Mrs West were both in poor physical health. Mrs West suffered from asthma and arthritis but was able to care for her husband who recently experienced a stroke and a leg injury. After an accident Mrs West was rushed to hospital. With her inability to return home, her husband was admitted on a trial basis into Elizabeth House, to be joined by his wife on her discharge from hospital. An attempt at rehabilitation proved fruitless.

The experience of being alone if one member entered hospital also tipped the balance in the admission to private care. Mrs Ester at Greenfields felt unable to continue living alone, particularly as her husband's chance of rehabilitation home after an amputation was very slim.

The competing demands of work, home and caring for a dependent relative proved too much for some families, to the extent that one daughter attempted suicide (see Chapter Six). Sometimes there were even competing dependencies and interests between different family or household members. One lady, Mrs Hawkins (Underwood) experienced a situation where her four daughters, all in their seventies, each cared for a physically sick husband, one of whom was in the terminal stages of cancer. An admission to hospital and then private care was the only option seen by this daughter to ease her load.

Unwilling families

With the strains on carers, it was not surprising that a group of relatives were more forceful and refused to continue or initiate involvement in caring for their elderly relative. However, only ten (5 per cent) of elderly residents experienced an unwillingness on the part of their families to care.

The different views of the care situation held by relatives and residents highlighted one of the difficulties in gauging the character of admission.

arranged by the ward sister and the manager of the private home who previously had visited the ward touting for business.

The residents were all well institutionalized for a variety of psychiatric and social reasons and it was this group who made up a proportion of 'young elderly' people moving into private residential care. Mrs Carton had been in hospital twelve years since the death of her husband; while another patient, Joan, had been institutionalized for forty years after giving birth to an illegitimate child.

2. Another group of six residents were rejected by other institutions in which they lived. Five of them had symptoms of advanced senile dementia, accompanied by psychiatric problems and very demanding and manipulative behaviour. The manager of the home described one lady:

> She is just pathetic - it's impossible to give 24-hour care and I can see why the other home got rid of her.

Another resident was described as having a 'dreadful past' as far as her psychiatric history was concerned - in and out of hospital with accopia and depression and living in appalling conditions.

3. For the third group, a local authority home was a real possibility, but the private sector provided a vacancy first.

> I just came in while I was waiting for a (local authority) home but there were never any vacancies so I stayed. If I'd followed the social worker's plan I'd have ended up in hospital. (Mrs Vickery)

> The situation was dire and she (mother) became hopeless. We couldn't wait for the GP to do anything so the welfare decided what to do in the end and we went ahead with the first vacancy. (Daughter of Mrs York)

Two other relatives chose this home in preference to a local authority one.

Elderly people who entered these three homes were very similar in profile to those confused elderly people entering local authority homes. This section demonstrated, however, that the private sector was more flexible and gave opportunity to those for whom local authority care may not have been a priority due to their location: that is, people not 'at risk' by virtue of being in hospital, or due to the support they already received through their family networks.

These three examples also show that mental deterioration alone was not significant as a single factor for entry into private residential care. Over three-quarters of the residents identified other specific reasons for entry into the private home, many of these factors were of social origin. Although physical and mental health problems dominated the background to admissions into private homes, social reasons were more prominent in directly leading to admission into the home.

home help and a laundry service, and supported family networks in their efforts to contain situations with very demented and often difficult people, many families could not sustain their commitment to care. Other families continued to struggle over a number of years and were often unable to recognise the 'breaking point' in terms of their own health as the following case study illustrates:

> She went into hospital after I broke my leg. It was up to me to set the discharge date. I just felt I couldn't cope any longer and I finally had to admit I had been struggling for a long time. (Husband of Mrs Anson)

In this case Mrs Anson returned home with increased support from the CPN and daily visits to the local psychiatric day hospital. Unfortunately, this did not abate her aggression, particularly toward her husband who was unable to 'maintain a life of his own' according to the CPN who initiated Mrs Anson's admission because Mr Anson was on the point of breakdown. The home owner reported that:

> Mr Anson found it hard to accept the situation but he decided there was no alternative.

In another instance the CPN was desperate to get the family to accept that their elderly relative needed residential care:

> Both son and stepson just couldn't see she was in desperate need. The situation got beyond them with the police and neighbours getting involved.

Another family resisted attempts to find a suitable vacancy as the following example portrayed:

> The CPN had to speak to me over and over again for a long time about this private home before I realised my mother's confusion wouldn't go away and would only get worse. At first we declined the vacancy - just didn't want her in a home and there was no way I would dump her although she's abused me all my life ... One month later we just had to accept another vacancy. (Daughter of Mrs Boyle)

Admission to this particular home often came after an admission to hospital where a psychiatric assessment took place. If support systems were evident, as in the case of Mr Anson, then in some instances there was a move back to the community prior to admission to Willow House.

The Suffolk. Three distinct groups of people entered this home through different channels.

1. With the re-organisation and closure of wards in the local psychiatric hospital a number of long-term psychiatric patients (7 out of 27) were 'rehabilitated' into the community; their route into the Suffolk being

(52 per cent), another home (16 per cent) or had received a package of care at home which had broken down (32 per cent). The majority of residents in each home had previously been assessed and admitted to psychiatric hospitals and therefore had contact with professionals - either social workers, community psychiatric nurses or psychiatrists who were influential in their movement through the process.

Examples could be found where psychiatrists suggested residential care or the social worker persuaded the family, near to breakdown, that they would benefit from such a move. This often resulted in a move directly into a private home, or a period at home with increased levels of support, the latter of which often broke down and necessitated a re-admission (Chapter 6).

Crabfield Hall. All residents at this home suffered from one of a variety of psychiatric states and were in advanced conditions of senile dementia. Depending on mental state, they presented different behavioral difficulties - loss of sexual inhibitions, delusions, eccentric behaviour and physical abuse, among others. As a result, many were unable to return to their previous setting in the community because of such disruptive and difficult behaviour. Mental disorders were of a severe nature - one resident suffered clinical depression with delusions about bodily functions; another, as a result of her senile dementia, lost all sexual inhibitions which made life impossible outside such an institution. Like a number of residents, these two women suffered long-standing problems which repeatedly required hospitalisation either as in-patients over a period of years or through treatment as out-patients with support from social workers and CPNs. The local psychiatric hospital was a filtering point in the process for four (60 per cent) of the interviewed residents who entered this home.

For residents with confusion, the role of the carer was paramount in supporting them in the community. Relatives often went to great lengths to hold difficult situations together and to mask problems caused by the elderly person's confusion. Their death often precipitated the move into hospital. On the other hand, parting with a wife or husband suffering with confusion was a traumatic event in itself for the carer as well as the resident as is illustrated below:

> We'd been married 53 years. Six years ago her memory started going, she then became difficult to handle and got progressively worse. It's awful as she's been a wonderful wife, cook and mother ... She used to say she hated me and often turned on me, but I didn't want her to go into a home. (Husband of Mrs Lowe)

> Her personality was fiercely dominating and she continued to rule the situation like a rod of iron. I lived nearby and as a result I suffered hell. (Grand-daughter of Mrs Waters)

Willow House. Similar people were found at Willow House, predominantly female residents suffering advanced states of senile dementia. The main difference was that most residents and their relatives had been supported in the community by the community psychiatric nursing service. Although CPNs arranged modest support systems, eg day care once or twice a week, contradiction in terms when cost-effectiveness and choice are in conflict and choice comes down to what the client can afford. How this area of effectiveness will be monitored is yet to be seen and will probably be governed by principles more akin to accountancy than social welfare.

As yet there is little knowledge as to who will control the budget and whether social workers are to take on the function of case management. If both are at the social worker level then it requires social workers to embrace a much broader conceptualisation of their role. They will have to understand various meanings and definitions of accountability to the agency and client; they will have to understand evaluative mechanisms for achieving effectiveness - oriented accountability and be able to collect and manage data for accountability (Moxley, 1989). They will also need to be aware of the potential conflict created in carrying out this function.

2. Direct service provision will be external. Thatcherite policy embodied wholeheartedly the mixed economy of welfare. The policy of privatization has pervaded every aspect of the welfare state, more than could have been imagined in the area of welfare for older people. Little of this move was based on sound researched evidence of the need for a shift in policy focus but was manouvered on ideological grounds.

Privatized provision has been pushed on the attractiveness of concepts such as choice, value for money and better quality to the service user. Yet since 1979 little research has been carried out on the private sector, it's effectiveness, the choice it affords it's customers and it's value for money. The research outlined in this book has shown that choice, for example, is far from the hands of the user. In other words, there are few indications that the private sector delivers what the Government intended. The Community Care Act has taken much for granted.

Policy is increasingly governed by the ideology of the free market, which in relation to older people means a shift to the private market away from state provision. In this arena the policy of pluralism is a euphemism for the selling off of state provision and moving welfare into the non-state sector.

Local Authorities are being forced to sell off their residential provision, because of the lack of capital funding made available to the state sector. This residualization of public sector services means a major shift in their role as providers of provision; what is even more radical is that Local Authorities are expected and have a statutory duty to promote the private and voluntary sectors of care. This is a major task as the domiciliary area of private care is barely existent. The experience gained in relation to the relationship with the private residential sector is of some use in this sense. Many mistakes were made which should not be repeated in the promotion of the private domiciliary arena. Again it is the less able older people who will experience the effects of privatization first.

State provision will increasingly be left as a second class provision, stigmatised and reserved for those with 'challenging behaviour'. In other words the rejects of the market system. Such a service is not likely to attract professionals who have experience of, and trained under a state system, underpinned by social work values and principles. Residential work with older people will be seen as committing professional suicide. The professionalism developed under the state system is not likely to be easily transferred to the private sector given the resistance and hesitation found among social workers in this research.

The shift in role to enabler rather than direct provider will have several consequences for the future of local authority social work. Local Authorities are equipping themselves as regulators and inspectors of the private sector. Policing the private sector has been the traditional role rather than one of befriending and promoting welfare in a competitive sector. To combine policing and befriending is a difficult if not impossible task (Chapter 1). Even within the public sector joint planning has been fraught with difficulties between NHS and SSD's (Audit Commission, 1986). The Community Care Act stresses the role of planning between sectors which will be an even bigger task. With no Government money ringfenced for this and the current dearth of private home care facilities will SSD's spend their energies in promoting this alternative sector? The planning task that lies ahead in the encouragement of the private sector to develop in an equitable fashion will not be easy. How extensive will such provision be when it exists, will it be geographically located to promote equal access for all older people and to what extent will it be financially beyond the reach of older people? A guarantee that older people in need will have stability and continuity in their care cannot be given as the vagaries of the market place take precedence over older people's welfare. Such dilemmas are hidden in the new Act.

For social workers they will need to gain an understanding of the problems and difficulties inherent in achieving interagency and interdisciplinary cooperation and coordination, difficulties around communication, and planning, monitoring and interpersonal areas of practice which this research highlights. The task facing social workers with older people in the 1990's, therefore, is developing an appropriate role for themselves in the private welfare market while grounding their practice firmly in social work values and principles and developing a system of accountability which doesn't lose sight of the needs of the client and their support system. Such is the challenge ahead.

Bibliography

Abrams, M. (1978) *Beyond three score years and ten: final report on a survey of the elderly*, Mitcham, Age Concern

Anderson, M. (1971) *Family structure in 19th century Lancashire* Cambridge, Cambridge University Press

Anderson, M. (1974) *Qualitative indicates of family change in the sociology of the family*, London, Penguin

Allen, I. (1983) *Short-stay residential care for the elderly* London, Policy Studies Institute

Archbishop of Canterbury (1985) *Faith in the city, a call for action by church and nation*, the report of the Archbishop of Canterbury's Commission on urban priority areas, London, Church Housing Publishing

Association of Directors of Social Services (1985) *Who goes where?* A profile of elderly people who have recently been admitted to residential homes, London, ADSS

Ackland, M. (1987) 'Privatisation: a look at some of the comparisons', *Social Work Today*, vol.19(9), p.19

Audit Commission for Local Authorities in England and Wales (1985) *Managing social services for the elderly more effectively*, London HMSO

Audit Commission for Local Authorities in England and Wales (1986) *Making a reality of community care*, London HMSO

Avebury, K. (1984) *Home life: a code of practice for residential care*, report of a working party, London, Centre for Policy on Ageing

Barclay Committee (1982) *Social workers: their role and tasks*, London Bedford Square Press/NCVO

Barnes, C.D. (1980) *The relentless tide: a study of admissions into homes for the elderly*, Guildford, Surrey County Council, Social Services Department

Bartlett, H & Brooke-Ross, R. (1986) 'Terms of a contract', *Community Care*,

no. 592, pp.14-16
Bartlett, H. & Challis, L. (1985) 'Constraints on care: supplementary benefit, the elderly and the private sector', *Social Services Research*, no. 5.
Bartlett, H. & Challis, L. (undated) *Private nursing homes for the elderly: a survey conducted in the south of England*, working paper no. 3, University of Bath, Centre for the Analysis of Social Policy
Bayley, M. (1973) *Mental handicap and community care*, London, Routledge & Kegan Paul
Bean, P. & McPherson, S. (eds) (1983) *Approaches to welfare*, London, Routledge & Kegan Paul
Bebbington, A.C. & Tong, M.S. (1983) 'Trends and changes in old people's homes: provision over twenty years', in Judge, K. and Sinclair, I. (edgs), *Residential care for elderly people*, London, HMSO
Beddoe, C. (1985a) quoted in Hemsley, J. 'A morally defensive stance', *Community Care*, no.590, pp.14-16
Beddoe, C. (1985b) 'The private sector is here to stay: a partnership must be forged', paper presented to the Social Care Association seminar 'Partners or competitors', Bloomsbury Crest Hotel, London
Beddoe, C. (1988) 'Future arrangements for private residential care: responses from the private sector', paper presented to the University of Keele/Polytechnic of North London conference 'The future of private residential care', 15 March, Connaught Hall, London
Berthoud, R. (ed) (1985) *Challenges to social policy*, Aldershot, Gower
Benson, S. (1987) 'Principle versus pragmatism?', *Community Care*, 15 January, no.644, pp.21-23
Bessell, B. (1983a) 'Bridges or Barriers?', *Community Care*, 25 February, p.24
Bessell, B. (1983b) 'In defence of the private sector', *Community Care*, 29 September, no. 481, pp.14-15
Beveridge, W. (1942) *Social insurance and allied services*, Cmnd.6404, London HMSO
Biggs, S. (1987a) 'Local authority registration staff and the boundary between public and private sector care', *Policy and Politics*, vol.15(4), pp.235-44
Biggs, S. (1987b) 'Quality of care and the growth of private sector welfare for old people', *Critical Social Policy*, vol.7(2), pp.74-82
Billis, D. (1973) 'Entry into residential care', *British Journal of Social Work*, 3(4), pp.447-71
Black, J., Bow, R., Burns, D., Critcher, C., Grant, G & Stockford D. (1983) *Social work in context: a comparative study of three social services teams*, London, Tavistock
Blaikie, A. & MacNicol, J. (1986) 'Towards an anatomy of ageism: society, social policy and the elderly between the wars', in Phillipson, C. Bernard, M & Strang, P (eds) *Dependency and independence*, London, Croom Helm
Bland, R. & Bland, R.E. (1983) 'Recent research in old people's homes: a review of the literature', *Research, Policy and Planning*, vol.1(1), pp.16-24
Bloomfield, J. (1986) 'Coventry's private care homes for elderly people', Social Services Research Department, Coventry Metropolitan Borough Council, pp.78-87
Blythe, R. (1981) *The view in winter*, London, Penguin
Booth, T. (1985) *Home truths: old people's homes and the outcome of care*, London, Gower

Booth, T. & Phillips, D. (1987) 'Group living in homes for the elderly: a comparative study of the outcome of care', *British Journal of Social Work*, 17(1), pp.1-20
Bosanquet, N. (1978) *A future for old age*, London, Temple Smith
Bowl, R. (1986) 'Social work with older people', in Phillipson, C. & Walker, A. *Ageing and social policy: a critical assessment*, Aldershot, Gower
Bradshaw, J. & Gibbs, I. (1987a) 'The problems with assessing the need for residential care', *Social Work Today*, August 10, vol.18(49), pp.12-13
Bradshaw, J. & Gibbs, I. (1987b) 'Supplementary benefit and residential care - assessment of needs and charges: Part B, the reasonableness of charges study', Social Policy Research Unit, University of York
Bradshaw, J. & Gibbs, I. (1988) *Public support for private residential care: studies in cash and care*, Aldershot, Gower
Brearley, C.P. (1975) *Social work, ageing and society*, London, Routledge & Kegan Paul
British Association of Social Workers (1977) 'Social work with the elderly: guidelines from BASW', *Social Work Today*, vol.8(27), pp.7-15
British Association of Social Workers (1984) 'Practice notes for social workers and registration officers working with the private and voluntary residential sectors', report of the project group on private and voluntary residential care, Birmingham, BASW
British Association of Social Workers (1986) 'The impact of the 1984 Registered Homes Act', Birmingham, BASW
Brocklehurst, J. Carty, M.H. & Robinson, J.M. (1978) 'Medical screening of old people accepted for residential care', *Lancet*, 2, 8081, pp.141-42
Bromley, D. (ed) (1984) *Gerontology: social and behavioural perspectives*, London, Croom Helm
Brooke-Ross, R. (1986a) 'Keeping the register up to date', *Social Services Insight*, vol.1(11), 15-22 March, p.13
Brooke-Ross, R. (1986b) 'Ways of keeping standards high' *Social Services Insight*, vol.1(14), 5-12 April, pp.14-15
Brooke-Ross, R. (1987) 'Registered homes and residents' well-being'. *Social Work Today*, vol.19(13), 23 November, pp.12-13
Brown, M. (1972) 'The development of local authority welfare services from 1948-1965 under Part III of the National Assistance Act 1948, PhD thesis, University of Manchester
Bull, D. & Wilding, P. (eds) (1983) *Thatcherism and the poor*, London, Child Poverty Action Group
Bulmer, M. (1986) *Neighbours: the work of Philip Abrams*, Cambridge, Cambridge University Press
Butler, A., Oldman, C. & Greves, J. (1983) *Sheltered housing: policy practice and the consumer*, London, Allen & Unwin
Bynum, W., Porter, R. & Shepherd, M. (eds) (1985) *The anatomony of madness: essays in the history of psychiatry*, (vol.2), London, Tavistock
Carson, D. (1985) 'Registering homes: another fine mess?' *Journal of Social Welfare Law*, March, pp.67-84
Cassam, E. (1987a) 'Home sweet home?', *Social Services Insight*, 1 May, vol.2(18), p.12-14
Cassam, E. (1987b) 'Can there be a partnership between the statutory and private sectors? - the Norfolk experience' in Lewis, B. et al, *Care and*

Control, discussion paper no.15, Policy Studies Institute, London
Central Council for the Education and Training in Social Work (1973() 'Social work: residential work is a part of social work', CCETSW paper no.3
Challis, D. & Davies, B. (1980) 'A new appraoch to community care for the elderly', *British Journal of Social Work*, vol.10(1), pp.1-18
Challis, D. & Davies, B. (1986) *Case management in community care, an evaluated experiment in the home care of the elderly*, Aldershot, Gower
Challis, L. (1985) 'Controlling for care: private and voluntary homes registration and inspection - a forgotten area of social work', *British Journal of Social Work*, vol.15(1), pp.43-56
Charlesworth, A. & Wilkin, D. (1982) 'Dependency among old people in geriatric wards, psychiatric wards and residential homes - 1977-81', Research Report No.6, Department of Psychiatry and Community Medicine, University of Manchester
Chronically Sick & Disabled Peoples Act (1972) London, HMSO
Churchill, J. (1985) 'Restricted by red tape', *Community Care*, no.577 29 August, pp.12-13
Clarke, M. (1982) 'Where is the community which cares?' *British Journal of Social Work*, vol.12, pp.453-69
Clarke, R. (1985) 'The last 10 years: a critical assessment of what "partnership" has meant in practice', paper presented to the Social Care Association seminar 'Partners or competitors?, Bloomsbury Crest Hotel, London
Cooper, M. (1985) 'The growth of private residential care in North East Essex - its impact on plans for local authority provision, Social Services Department, Essex County Council
Clough, R. (1981) *Old age homes*, London, Allen & Unwin
Clough, R. & Wigg, M. (1982) 'Workhouse revisited' *Social Work Today*, 23 February, vol.13(24), p.17
Clough, R. (1987) 'Independent review of residential care for the elderly within the London Borough of Camden', London Borough of Camden
Cumming, E.M. & Henry, W.E. (1961) *Growing old: the process of disengagement*, New York, Basic Books
Curnock, K. & Hardiker, P. (1979) *Towards practice theory*, London, Routledge & Kegan Paul
Darton, R. (1986) *Survey of residential accommodation for the elderly, 1981*, Personal Social Services Research Unit, University of Kent
Darton, R. & McCoy, P. (1981) 'Survey of residential accommodation for the elderly', Claring House for Local Authority Social Services, Research Report No.2, pp.23-44
Davidson, N. (1983) 'On the waterfront', *Social Work Today*, vol.15(4), pp.4-5
Davies, B. (1986) 'The production of welfare approach', discussion paper no.400, Personal Social Services Research Unit, University of Kent
Davies, B. & Challis, D. (1986) *Matching resources to need in community care*, Aldershot, Gower
Davies, B. & Knapp, M. (1981) *Old people's homes and the production of welfare*, London Routledge & Kegan Paul
Davies, M. (1979) 'Swopping the old around', *Community Care*, 18 October, no.286, pp16-17
Davies, M. (1985) *The essential social worker: a guide to positive practice*,

(second edition), Aldershot, Gower
Day, P. (1985) 'Regulating the private sector of welfare', *Political Quarterly*, vol.56(3), pp.282-85
Department of Health (1989) 'Residential accommodation statistics, Part A, B and E, (RAC 5), Department of Health: Statistics and Research, London HMSO
Department of Health and Social Security (1972) 'Local Government Act: Section 195', London, HMSO
Department of Health and Social Security (1976) 'Priorities in the health and personal social services', consultative document, London, HMSO
Department of Health and Social Security (1977) 'The Way Forward', London, HMSO
Department of Health and social Security (1978) 'A happier old age: a discussion document, London, HMSO
Department of Health and Social Security (1981a) 'Growing older', Cmnd. 8173, London HMSO
Department of Health and Social Security (1981b) 'Care in action: a handbook of policies and priorities for the health and social services in England', London, HMSO
Department of Health and Social Security (1983) 'Social security statistics', London, HMSO
Department of Health and Social Security (1987a) *Inspection of the implementation of the 1984 Registered Homes Act*, report of the Social Services Inspectorate, London, HMSO
Department of Health and Social Security (1987b) 'Public Support for residential care', report of the Joint Central and Local Government Working Party (The Firth Report), London, HMSO
Department of Health and Social Security (1987c) 'Health and personal social services statistics for England', (1987 edition), London, HMSO
Department of Health and Social Security (1988) 'Community care: agenda for action, (Griffiths Report), report to the Secretary of State for Social Services, London HMSO
Department of Health and Social Security (1990) Caring for People 'Community Care and Beyond', London, HMSO
Department of Health and Social Security (1991) 'Implementing Community Care. Purchaser, Commissioner & Provider Roles', London, HMSO
Department of Social Security & the Central Office of Information (1989) 'Social security benefit rates', leaflet NI 196 from April 1989, London HMSO
Dingwell, R., Heath, C., Reid, M. & Stacey, M. (eds) (1983) *Health care and health knowledge*, London, Croom Helm
Dexter, M. & Harbert, W. (1983) *The home help service*, London, Tavistock
Etherington, S. (1985) 'Private care is a public concern', *Social Work Today*, vol.15(8), 25 October
Equal Opportunities Commission (1982) *Caring for the elderly and handicapped: community care policies and women's lives*, Manchester
Ermisch, J. (1983) *The political economy of demographic change*, London, Heinemann
Ernst & Whinney Ltd. (1986) 'Survey of private and voluntary residential and nursing homes for the DHSS', Bicester, Ernst & Whinney

Evandrou, M., Arber, S., Dale, A. & Gilbert, N. (1986) 'Who cares for the elderly? Family care provision and receipt of statutory services', in Phillipson, C., Barnard, M. & Strang, P. (eds), *Dependency and interdependency in old age: theoretical perspectives and policy Alternatives*, London, Croom Helm

Fennell, G. (1986) *Anchor's older people: what do they think?*, Oxford, Anchor Housing Association

Finch, J. & Groves, D. (1980) 'Community care and the family: a case for equal opportunities', *Journal of Social Policy*, vol.9(4), pp.487-511

Finch, J. & Groves, D. (eds) (1983) *A labour of love: women, work and caring*, London, Routledge & Kegan, Paul

Fisher, M. (1991) 'Defining the practice content of Case Management' *in Social Work & Social Sciences Review*, vol 2(3) 1990-91, London, Whiting & Birch

Fisk, M. (1986) *Independence and the elderly*, London, Croom Helm

Gibbs, I. & Bradshaw, J. (1988) 'Needs must fit', *Social Services Insight*, 24 July, vol.2(30), p.17-19

Gibbs, I. & Bradshaw, J. (1988) 'Dependency and its relationship to the assessment of care needs of elderly people', *British Journal of Social Work*, vol.18, pp.577-92

Gill, P. (1988) *Residential care for elderly people*, Social Work Monographs, No.67, School of Economic and Social Studies, University of East Anglia

Glaser, B. & Strauss, A. (1967) *The discovery of grounded theory*, Chicago, Alpine Publishing

Glendenning, F. (ed) (1981) *Care in the community: recent research and the current projects*, Stoke on Trent, Beth Johnson Foundation in association with Age Concern and University of Keele

Godlove, C., Richard, L. & Rodwell, G. (1982) *Time for action*: an observation study of elderly people in four different care environments, University of Sheffield, Joint Unit for Social Services Research

Goffman, E. (1961) *Asylum: essays on the social situation of mental patients and other inmates*, New York, Penguin

Goldberg, E.M. (1970) *Helping the Aged*, London, Allen & Unwin

Goldberg, E.M. et al (1978) 'Towards accountability in social work: long-term social work in an area office', *British Journal of Social Work*, vol.8(3), pp.253-87

Goldberg, E,M. & Connelly, N. (1982) *The effectiveness of social care for the elderly*, London, Heinemann

Goldberg, E.M. & Hatch, S. (eds) (1981) *A new look at the personal social services*, discussion paper no. 4, Policy Studies Institute, London

Goldberg, E.M. & Warburton, W.R. (1979) *Ends and means in social work: the development and and outcome of a case review sytem*, London, Allen & Unwin

Golding, P. (1983) 'Rethinking commonsense about social policy', in Bull, D. & Wilding, P. (eds), *Thatcherism and the poor*, London, Child Poverty Action Group

Greengross, S. (1982) 'Caring for the carers', in Glendenning, F. (ed) *Care in the community: recent research and current projects*, Stoke on Trent, Beth Johnson Foundation

Grindod, N., Leigh, A. & Smith, S. (1987) 'Private care, public concern', *Community Care*, 1 January, no.642, pp.18-19 Hadley, R. (1981) 'Social services departments and the community' in Goldberg, E.M. & Hatch, S. (eds), *A new look at the personal social services*, London, Policy Studies Institute

Harbert, W.B. (1980) 'Admissions to homes for the elderly - a survey and assessment of alternatives', Avon County Council, Social Services Department

Harris, A. (1968) *The social welfare of the elderly*, London, HMSO

Harris, D. & Hyland, J. (1979) *Rights in residence*, London, Residential Care Association

Health Advisory Service (1983) *The rising tide: developing services for mental illness in old age*, London, Health Advisory Service

Hemsley, J. (185) 'A morally defensive stance?', *Community Care*, 12 December, no.590 pp.14-16

Henderson, J. (1986) 'By the community: an ideological response to the crisis in the welfare state?, in Phillipson, C., Barnard, M. & Strang, P. (eds) *Dependency and interdependency in old age:, theoretical perspectives and policy alternatives*, London, Croom Helm

Henwood, M. & Wicks, N. (1986) 'Benefit or burden?: the objectives and impact of child support', occasional paper no. 3, London, Family Policy Studies Centre

Higgins, J. (1985) 'Homing in on problems of care for the elderly', *Health & Social Service Journal*, 3 January, no.6, pp.12-13

Hitch, D. & Simpson, A. (1972) 'An attempt to assess a new design in residential homes for the elderly', *British Journal of Social Work*, vol.2(4), pp.481-501

House of Commons (1986) *Hansard*, 27 March, vol.123, cols.1135a-1136, London, HMSO

Howe, D. (1979) 'Agency function and social work principles', *British Journal of Social Work*, vol.9(10), pp.29-49

Howe, D. (1980) 'Divisions of labour in the area teams of social services departments', *Social Policy and Administration*, vol.14(2), pp.133-50

Hoyland, P. (1986) '"Wide abuse" in private homes for the elderly', *Guardian*, 29 April, p.3

Hughes, B. & Wilkin, D. (1980) 'Residential care of the elderly: a review of the literature', research report no.2, University of Manchester, Psychogeriatric Unit

Hunt, A. (1970) *The home help service in England and Wales*, London, HMSO

Hunt, A. (1978) *The elderly at home*: a study of people aged 65 and over living in the community in England in 1976, London, OPCS, HMSO

Jahoda, M., Deutsch, M. & Cook, S.W. (eds) (1951) *Research methods in social relations*, New York, Dryden Press

Jack, R. (1991) Social Services, Social Policy & the Ageing Population 1970-1990 *unpublished paper*, UEA Norwich

Jerrome, D. (ed) (1983) *Ageing in modern society*, London, Croom Helm

Johnson, M. (1984) 'Privatising residential care - a review of changing practice and policy', in Laming, H. (ed), *Residential care for the elderly: present problems and future issues*, London, Policy Studies Institute

Johnson, M. (1983) 'Controlling the cottage industry', *Community Care*, 25 August, no.476, p.16

Jolly, A. (9186) 'Private's progress', *Community Care*, 29 May no.613 pp.18-19

Jones, K. (1972) 'The 24 steps: an analysis of institutional admission procedures', *Sociology*, vol.6, p.407

Judge, K. (1982) 'The public purchase of social care', *Policy and Politics*, Vol.10(4), pp.397-417

Judge, K. (1985) 'Value for moey in the private residential care industry: a comparative analysis of variations in charges and costs in British residential homes for the elderly', discussion paper no. 394, Personal Social Services Research Unit, University of Kent, prepared for a joint meeting of Nordic HESG and UK HESG, Vadstena, Sweden

Judge, K. & Knapp, M. (1985) 'Efficiency in the production of welfare: the public and private sectors compared', in Klein, R. and O'Higgins, M. (eds), *The future of welfare*, Oxford, Basil Blackwell

Judge, K., Knapp, M. & Smith, J. (1986) 'The comparative costs of public and private residential homes for the elderly', chapter 10 in Judge, K. and Sinclair, I. (eds), *Residential care for elderly people*, London, HMSO

Judge, K. & Sinclair, I. (eds) (1986) *Residential care for elderly people: research contributions to the development of policy and practice*, London, HMSO

Judge, K., Smith, J. & Taylor-Gooby, P. (1983) 'Public opinion and the privatisation of welfare: some theoretical implications', *Journal of Social Policy*, vol.12(4), pp.469-90

Kamerman, S.B. & Kahn, A.J. (eds) (1978) *Family policy, government and families in 14 countries*, New York, Columbia University Press

Kay, N. (1897) 'Firth: questions that need asking', *Social Services Insight*, vol.2(34), 21 August, p.2.

Kellaher, L., Peace, S., Weaver, T. & Willcoks, D. (1988) *Coming to terms with the private sector* - regulating practice for residential care homes and elderly people, Centre for Environmental Social Studies in Ageing, Polytechnic of North London

Klein, R. & O'Higginns, M. (eds) (1985) *The future of welfare*, Oxford, Basil Blackwell

Knapp, M.R.J. (1984) *The economics of social care*, London, Macmillan

Labour Party (1988) 'A collective pathway to individual freedom', *Guardian*, 6 February, p.14

Laing, W. & Buisson, L. (1985) 'Care of elderly people: the market for residential and nursing homes in Britain', London, Health Sector Consultancy

Laming, H. (ed) (1984) *Residential care for the elderly: present problems and future issues*, London, Policy Studies Institute

Land, H. (1978) 'Who cares for the family?', *Journal of Social Policy*, Vol.7(3), pp.357-84

Land, H. & Parker, R. (1978) 'Implicit and reluctant family policy - United Kingdom', in Kamerman, S.B. and Kahn, A.J. (eds), *Family policy: government and families in 14 countries*, New York, Columbia University Press

Larder, D., Day, P. & Klein, R. (1986) 'Institutional care for the elderly: the geographical distribution of the public/private mix in England', Social Policy Papers No.10, University of Bath

Leat, D. (1986) 'Privatisation and voluntarization', *Quarterly Journal of Social Affairs*, vol.2(3), pp.285-320

Le Grand, J. (1982) *The strategy of equality*, London, Allen & Unwin

Le Grand, J. & Robinson, R. (eds) (1984) *Privatisation and the welfare state*, London, Allen & Unwin
Leonard, P. (1982) Editor's introduction in Phillipson, C. *Capitalism and the construction of old age*, London, Macmillan
Lewis, B. et al (1987) *Care and control: personal social services and the private sector*, discussion paper no.15, London, Policy Studies Institute
Lipman, A. & Slater, R. (1977) 'Homes for old people: towards a positive environment', *The Gerontologist*, vol.17(2), pp.146-56
Loney, M. et al (eds) (1987), *The state or the market*, London, Sage
Loney, M., Bocock, R., Clarke, J., Cochrane, A., Graham, P. & Wilson, M. (eds) (1987) *The state or the market: politics and welfare in contemporary Britain*, London, Sage
Mabon, G. (1989) 'A view from the private sector', in Philpot, T. (ed), *The residential opportunity: the Wagner report and after*, Wallington, Community Care/Reed Business Publishing
MacLennan, W.J., Isles, F.E., McDougall, S. & Keddie, E. (1984) 'Medical and social factors influencing admission to residential care', *British Medical Journal*, 288,6418, pp.701-03
MacPherson, I., Hunter, D.J. & McKeganey, N.P. (1988) 'Interviewing elderly people: some problems and challenges', *Research and Policy Planning*, vol.5(2), pp.13-18
Marshall, T.H. (1965) *Social policy*, London, Hutchinson University Library
Maynard, A. (1987) 'Towards an efficient marker in the care of the elderly', unpublished paper to British Society of Gerontology symposium, 'Policies for elderly people', 17 October, London
McCoy, P. (1983) 'Short-term residential care for elderly people: an answer to growing older', in Jerrome, D. (ed), *Ageing in modern society,* London, Croom Helm
McCoy, P. (1984) 'Private lives', in Bromley, D. (ed) *Gerontology: social and behavioural perspectives*, London, Croom Helm
McCoy, P. (1986) 'Ten years after the ten year plan: 1984 or homage to Catatonia?, unpublished dissertation for MA in Social Services Planning Department of Sociology, University of Essex
McIntyre, S. (1977) 'Old age as a social problem', in Dingwall, R., Heath, C., Reid, M. & Stacy, M. (eds) *Health care and health knowledge*, London, Croom Helm
McKenzie, S. & Baldock, P. (1981) 'The contribution of the private and voluntary sector to the residential care of the elderly: a study in Suffolk', unpublished paper, Social Work Service, London North Region
Meacher, M. (1972) *Taken for a ride:*, London, Longman
Means, R. & Smith R. (1983) 'From public assistance institutions to "sunshine" hotels: changing state perceptions about residential care for elderly people', *Ageing and Society*, vol.3(2), pp.157-81
Means, R. & Smith, R. (1985) *The development of welfare services for elderly people*, London, Croom Helm
Midwinter, E. (1986) *Caring for cash: the value of private domiciliary care*, London, Centre for Policy on Ageing
Miller, E.J. & Gwynne, G.V. (1972) *A life apart*, London, Tavistock
Minford, P. (1984) *State expenditure: a study in waste*, London, Instiitute of Economic Affairs

Minford, P. (1987) 'The role of the social services: a view from the New Right', in Loney, M. et al (eds), *The state or the market*, London, Sage
Ministry of Health (1948) *National Assistance Act 1948*, circular 87/48, London, HMSO
Mitchell, S. & Earwicker, J. (1982) 'Getting people placed: allocating places in residential homes - an analysis of the decision process', London Borough of Hammersmith and Fulham
Moore, J. (1988) 'Elderly people are usually upwardly mobile', *Social Work Today*, 4 August, vol.19(48), p.5.
Moroney, R.M. (1976) *The family and the state: considerations for social policy*, London Longmans
Morris, P. (1986) 'BASW backs move towards private care', *Community Care*, 13 March, no.602, p.4
Moxley, (1989) *The Practice of Case Management*, London, Sage
Murray, N. (1984) 'Privates on parade', *Community Care*, 8 March, no.502, pp.18-21
National Union of Public Employees (1986) 'The realities of home life', report of a research project commissioned by the West Midlands County Council Economic Development Unit, NUPE/WMCC
Neill, J. (1982) 'Some variations in policy and procedure relating to Part III applications in the GLC area', *British Journal of Social Work*, 12, pp.229-46
Neill, J., Sinclair, I., Gorback, P. & Williams, J. (1988) *A need for care: study of elderly applicants for local authority residential care*, Aldershot, Gower
Nissel, M. & Bonnerjea, L. (1982) *Family care of the handicapped elderly: who pays*, London, Policy Studies Institute
Norfolk County Council, (1985) 'Registration, inspection and professional support of private and voluntary residentil care homes: the Norfolk model', Norfolk County Council, Social Services Department
Norfolk County Council, (1986) 'Report of registered homes tribunal', decision of the tribunal held at County, Hall, Norwich on 14-15 January in the appeal of Mr & Mrs Swain (appellants and Norfolk County Council (respondent)
Norman, A. (1980) *Rights and risks*, London, Centre for Policy on Ageing.
Norton, A., Stoten, B. & Taylor, H. (1986) *Councils for care: planning a local government strategy for older people*, Policy Studies in Ageing No.5, London, Centre for Policy on Ageing
Nuffield Foundation (1947) *Old people*, report of a survey committee on the problems of ageing and the care of old people under the chairmanship of Seebohm Rowntree
Office of Population Census Surveys (1971) *Census 1971: GB non-private households*, London, HMSO
Office of Population Census Surveys (1980) *Classification of occupations*, London, HMSO
Office of Population Census Surveys (1981) *Census 1981: GB, sex, age and marital condition*, London, HMSO
Office of Population Census Surveys (1983) *Census 1981: persons of pensionable age*, London, HMSO
Office of Population Census Surveys (1981) 'Population projections: 1981-2021', London, HMSO

Office of Population Census Surveys (1987) 'Monthly digest of statistics', June, London, HMSO
Ovenstone, I.M.K. & Bean, P.T.A. (1981) 'A medical, social assessment of admissions to old people's homes in Nottingham', *British Journal of Psychiatry*, 139, pp.226-29
Papadakis, E. & Taylor-Gooby, P. (1987) *The private provision of public welfare: state, market and community*, Sussex, Wheatsheaf Books
Parkes, C.M. (172) *Bereavement: studies of grief in adult life*, London, Tavistock Publications
Parsons, M. (1986) 'The battle of Leicester', *This Caring Concern*, April, no.1, p.32
Paterson, L. (1978) 'A suitable case for care: the selection of residents for old people's homes', *Health & Social Service Journal*, 88(4580), pp.E1-E4
Peace, S.M. (1986) 'The forgotten female: social policy and older women, in Phillipson, C. & Walker, A., *Ageing and social policy*, Aldershot, Gower
Peace, S.M. (1979) *The quality of life of the elderly in residential care*, Research Report No.1, Survey Research Unit, Polytechnic of North London
Peace, S.M. & Harding, S.D. (1980) 'The Haringay group - living evaluation project', Research Report No.2, Survey Research Unit, Polytechnic of North London
Peacock, A.T. & Wiseman, J. (1961) *The growth of public expenditure in the U.K.*, Oxford, Oxford University Press
Peaker, C. (1986) 'The crisis in residential care', London, National Council for Voluntary Organisations
Phillips, D. & Vincent, J. (1986a) 'Petit bourgeois care: private residential care for the elderly', *Politics and Policy*, vol.14(2), pp/189-208
Phillips, D. & Vincent J. (1986b) 'Private residential accommodation for the elderly: geographical aspects of developments in Devon', *Transcripts of the Institute of British Geographers*, vol.11, pp.155-73
Phillips, D., Vincent, J. & Blacksell, S. (1988) *Home from home?* Private residential care for elderly people', Joint Unit for Social Services Research, University of Sheffield
Phillipson, C. (1982) *Capitalism and the construction of old age*, London, Macmillan
Phillipson, C. (1988) 'Planning for community care: facts and fallacies in the Griffiths Report', Working paper no.1, Centre for Social Gerontology, University of Keele
Phillipson, C., Barnard, M. & Strang, P. (1986) *Dependency and interdependency in old age: theoretical perspectives and policy alternatives*, London, Croom Helm
Phillipson, C. & Walker, A. 1986) *Ageing and social policy: a critical assessment*, Aldershot, Gower
Philpot, T. (ed) (189) *The residential opportunity: the Wagner report and after*, Wallington, Community Care/Reed Business Publishing
Pinker, R. (1983) 'Social welfare and the education of social workers', in Bean, P. & McPherson, S. (eds), *Approaches to welfare*, London, Routledge & Kegan Paul
Plank, D. (1977) 'Caring for the elderly: report of a study of various means of caring for dependent elderly people in 8 London Boroughs', Greater London Council

Pope, P. (1978) 'Admissions to residential homes for the elderly', *Social Work Today*, vol.9(4), pp.12-16
Queshri, H. & Walker, A. (1986) *The caring relationship: elderly people and their families*, London, Macmillan
Reid, J.W. & Epstein, L. (1972) *Task centred casework*, New York, Columbia University Press
Registered Homes Act (1980) London, HMSO
Registered Homes Act (1984) London, HMSO
Robb, B. (1967) *Sans everything: a case to answer*, London, Nelson
Robinson, R. (1986) 'Restructuring the welfare state: an analysis of public expenditure 1979/80-1984-85', *Journal of Social Policy*, vol.15(1), pp.1-21
Room, G. (1979) *The sociology of welfare*, Oxford, Blackwell
Rose, M.E. (1972) *The relief of poverty: 1834-1914*, London, Macmillan
Rosser, C. & Harris, C. ('965) *The family and social change*, London, Routledge & Kegan Paul
Rossiter, C. & Wicks, M. (1982) *Crisis or challenge? Family care, elderly people and social policy*, London, Study Commission on the Family
Rowlings, C. (1981) *Social work with elderly people*, London, Allen & Unwin
Rowntree, B.S. (1901) *Poverty: a study of town life*, London, Macmillan
Royal Commission on the Poor Laws and the Relief of Distress 1909) 'Majority and minority reports', London, HMSO
Royal Commission on the Population (1949) Cmnd. 7695, London, HMSO
Salvage, A. (1988) 'Attitutdes of the over 75's to Health and Social Services: Final Report', Research Team for the Care of the Elderly, College of Medicine, University of Wales
Sainsbury, E. (1981) 'Sharing in welfare: community resources and the work of area teams', *Social Work Service*, no.27, pp.11-17
Seebohm Committee (1968) *Report of the committee on local authority and allied personal social services*, London, HMSO
Seldon, A. (1981) 'Wither the welfare state', Occasional Paper No.60, London, Institute of Economic Affairs
Shanas, E., Townsend, P., Wedderburn, D., Henning, F., Millhof, P. & Stehouwer, J. (1968) *Old people in three industrial societies*, London, Routledge & Kegan Paul
Shaw, I. & Walton, R. (1979) 'Transitions to residence in homes for the elderly', in Harris, D. and Hyland, J. (eds), *Rights in residence*, London, Residential Care Association
Sheldon, J. (1948) *The social medicine of old age*, London, Oxford University Press
Sinclair, I. (1986) 'The residents: characteristics and reasons for admission', in Judge, K. and Sinclair, I. (eds), *Residential care for elderly people*, London, HMSO
Sinclair, I. (ed) (1988) *Residential care: the research reviewed*, literature survey commissioned by the independent review of residential care chaired by Lady Wagner, London, HMSO
Sinclair, I., Stanforth, L. & O'Conner, P. (1988) 'Factors preciting admission of elderly people to local authority residentical care', *British Journal of Social Work*, vol.18(3), pp.251-69
Smith, R.G. & Lowther, C.P. (1976) 'Follow-up study of two hundred admissions to a residential home', *Age & Ageing*, vol.5, pp.176-80

Stevenson, O. & Parsloe, P. (1978) *Social services teams: the practitioner's view*, London HMSO
Suffolk County Council (1986a) 'Residential and day care services for elderly people', Suffolk County Council, Social Services Department
Suffolk County Council (1986b) 'Quarterly trends: Suffolk' no.17, June, 1986 Suffolk County Council, Social Services Department, Research and Planning Section
Taft, J. (ed) (1944) *A functional approach to family casework*, Pennsylvania, University of Pennsylvania Press
Taylor-Gooby, P. (1987) 'Welfare attitudes: clevage, consensus and citizenship', *Quarterly Journal of Social Affairs*, vol.3(2), p.57
Taylor-Gooby, P. & Dale, J. (1981) *Social theories and social welfare*, London, Edward Arnold
Thatcher, M. *Hansard*, vol.655, cols.1161-62
Thatcher, M. (1977) 'The healthy society', in *Let our children grow tall: selected speeches 1975-77*, London, Centre for Policy Studies
Thomson, D. (1983) 'Workhouse to nursing home: residential care of elderly people in England since 1840', *Ageing and Society*, vol13.(1), pp.43-69
Thomson, D. (1984) 'The decline of social welfare: falling state support for the elderly since early Victorian times', *Ageing and Society*, vol.4, pp.451-82
Tinker, A. (1981) *The elderly in modern society*, Essex, Longman
Tinker, A. (1984) *Staying at home: helping elderly people*, London, HMSO
Titmuss, R. (ed) (1958) *Essays on the welfare state* (second edition), London, Unwin University Books
Titmuss, R., Able-Smith, B. & Titmuss, K. (1974) *Social policy: an introduction*, London, Allen & Unwin
Tobin, S. & Lieberman, M. (1976) *Last home for the aged*, London, Jossey-Bass
Townsend, P. (1962) *The last refuge*, London, Routledge & Kegan Paul
Townsend, P. (1963) *The family life of old people*, Harmondsworth, Penguin
Townsend, P. & Wedderburn, D. (1965) *The aged in the welfare state*, London, Bell
Vickers, J. & Yarrow, G. (1985) *Privatisation: an economic analysis*, Cambridge, Mass, London, MIT Press
Vincent, J., Tibbenham, A. & Phillips, D. (1987) 'Choice in residential care: myths and realities', *Journal of Social Policy*, vol.16(4), pp.435-60
Vladeck, B.C. (1980) *Unloving care: the nursing home tragedy*, New York, Basic Books
Wade, B., Sawyer, L. & Bell, J. (1983) *Dependency with dignity: different care provisions for the elderly*, occasional papers on social administration, no.68, London, Bedford Square Press/NCVO
Wagner, G. (1988) *Residential care: a positive choice*, report of the independent review of residential care, London, HMSO
Walker, A. (1980) 'The social creation of poverty and dependency in old age', *Journal of Social Policy*, vol.9(1), pp.45-75
Walker, A. (1982) *Community care: the family, the state and the social policy*, Oxford, Roberts
Walker, A. (1985) 'The care gap: how can local authorities meet the needs of the elderly?', London, Local Government Information Unit
Walker, A. (1986) 'The politics of ageing in Britain', in Phillipson, C., Bernard, M. & Strang, P. (eds), *Dependency and interdependency in old age:*

theoretical perspectives and policy alternatives, London, Croom Helm
Walker, A. (1987) 'The social construction of dependency in old age', in Loney, M. et al (eds). *The state or the market*, London, Sage
Walker, A. (1988) 'Dependent relativities', *The Times Higher Education Supplement*, 22 April, p.17
Walker, C. & Walker, A. (1987) 'The growing divide', *Community Care'*, 2 July, no.667 pp.24-25
Wall, R. (1984) 'Residential isolation of the elderly: a comparison over time', *Ageing and Society*, vol.4(4), pp.483-503
Walton, J.K. (1985) 'Casting out and bringing back in Victorian England. Pauper lunatics, 1840-70', in Bynum, W.F., Porter, R. & Shepherd, M. (eds), *The anatomy of madness: essays in the history of psychiatry*, (vol.2), London, Tavistock
Walton, R. & Elliot, D. (eds) (1980) *Residential care: a reader in current theory and practice*, Oxford, Pergamon Press
Ward, L. (1980) 'The social work task inresidential care', in Walton, R. and Elliot, D. (eds), *Residential care: a reader in current theory and practice*, Oxford, Pergamon Press
Weale, A. (1983) *Political theory and social policy*, London, Macmillan
Weaver, T., Willcocks, D. & Kellaher, L. (1985a) *The pursuit of profit and care: patterns and processes in private residential homes for old people*, Centre for Environmental and Social Studies in Ageing, Polytechnic of North London
Weaver, T., Willcocks, D. & Kellaher, L. (1985b) *The business of care: a study of private residential homes for old people*, report no.1, Centre for Environmental and Social Studies, Polytechnic of North London
Webb, A. (1985) 'Alternative futures for social policy and state welfare', chapter 2 in Berthoud, R. (ed), *Challenges to social policy*, Alershot, Gower
Weir, S. & Simpson, R. (1980) 'Are the local authority social services being bled dry?', *New Society Survey*, p.62, New Society
Wenger, C.G. (1984) *The supportive network: coping with old age*, London, Allen & Unwin
West, P. (1984) 'The family, the welfare state and community care: political rhetoric and public attitudes', *Journal of Social Policy*, vol.13(4), pp.417-46
West, P., Illsley, R. & Kelman, K. (1984) 'Public preference for the care of dependency groups', *Social Science and Medicine*, vol.18(4). pp.287-95
White, J., Yeates, A. & Skipworth, G. (1974) *Tables for statisticians*, (second edition), Teeside Polytechnic, Cheltenham, Thornes
Wicks, M. (1978) *Old and cold*, London, Heineman
Wicks, M. (1982) 'Community care and elderly people', in Walker, A. (ed), *Community care: the family, the state and social policy*, Oxford, Blackwell
Wicks, M. (1987a) 'Family matters and public policy', in Loney, M. et al (eds), *The state or the market*, London, Sage
Wicks, M. (1987b) 'Shaping the state', *Social Services Insight*, 20 February, pp.22-24
Wilding, G.P. (1983) 'The evolution of social administration', in Bean, P. & McPherson, *Approaches to welfare*, London, Routledge & Kegan Paul
Wilkin, D. & Jolley, D. (1979) *Behavioural problems among old people in geriatric wards, psychogeriatric wards and residential homes*, 1976-78, Research Report, No. 1, Psychogeriatric Unit, University of South Manchester

Willocks, D., Peace, S., Kellaher, L with Ring, A. (1982) *The residential life of old people: a study in 100 local authority old peoples' homes*, vol.1, research report no.12, Survey Research Unit, Polytechnic of North London

Willcocks, D., Peace, S. & Kellaher, L. (1987) *Private lives in public places: a research-based critique of residential life in local authority old peoples' homes*, London, Tavistock

Williams, G. (1988) 'Private sector provision of sheltered housing: policy impacts and issues', paper to the British Society of Gerontology annual conference (September), University of Swansea

Wistow, G. (1987a) 'Increasing private provision of social care: implications for policy, in Lewis, B. et al, *Care and control*, London, Policy Studies Institute

Wistow, G. (1987b) 'Tying down the private sector', *Social Services Insight*, 29 May, vol.2(22), pp.14-16

Wright, F. (1983) 'Single carers: employment, housework and caring', in Finch, J & Groves, D. (eds), *A labour of love: women, work and caring*, London, Routledge & Kegan Paul

Young, M & Willmott, P. (1957) *Family and kinship in East London*, London, Penguin Books

Name index

Abrams, M. 8,224
Ackland, M. 40
Association of Directors of Social Services 133
Allen, I. 23
Anderson, M. 4,9
Arber, S. 11
Archbishop of Canterbury 39

Baldock, P. 51
Barclay, P. 12,15-17
Barnes, C.D. 28
Bartlett, H. & Challis L. 34,45
Bayley, M. 11
Bean, P. & Ovenstone 26,177
Bebbington, A.C. & Tong, M.S. 30
Beddoe, C. 41,42,45
Bell, J. 67
Benson, S. 44
Bessell, B. 37,38,43,44,110
Biggs, S. 38,43
Billis, D. 30
Black, J. 14-17
Blacksell, S. 36,38,45,78
Blaikie, A. & MacNicol, J. 3
Bland, R. & Bland, R.E. 68
Bloomfield, J. 98
Blythe, R. 8
Bonnerjea, L. 10,12
Booth, T. 25,66,67,85,88, 101,102,168
Bosanquet, N. 39
Bowl, R. 16
Bradshaw, J & Gibbs,I. 26,29,34, 44,45,98,99,190,237
Brearley, C.P. 14,27
Brocklehurst, J. 26
Brooke-Ross, R. 41,43
Brown, M. 22
Buisson, L. 34
Bull, D. & Wilding, P. 7
Bulmer, M. 11

Carson, D. 41
Cassam, E. 41,42
Challis, D., Challis, L. & Davies, B. 5,16,23,240
Churchill, J. 42
Clarke, J. 11,43
Clough, R. 30,40
Connelly, N. 17
Cooper, M. 28

Cumming, E.M. & Henry, W.E. 8
Curnock, K. & Hardiker, P. 25

Dale, A. 11
Darton, R. 23,51
Davidson, N. 35
Day, P. 32,37
Dexter, M. & Herbert, W. 17

Earwicker, J. 28-30
Epstein, L. 15
Ermisch, J. 5
Ernst & Whinney Ltd. 34
Etherington, S. 42
Evandrou, M. 11

Fennell, G. 68
Finch, J. & Groves, D. 10,193
Gibbs, I. & Bradshaw, J. 26,29, 34,44,45,98,99,190,237
Gilbert, N. 11
Gill, P. 19,32,23
Glaser, B. & Strauss, A. 62
Glendenning, F. 16
Goffman, E. 21,26,85
Goldberg, E.M. 14-17
Golding, P. 7,35
Greengross, S. 9
Grindod, N. 41
Groves, D. 10,193
Gwynne, G.V. 21,27

Hadley, R. 17,22
Hall, 68
Hamblin, 68
Hardiker, P. 25
Harris, C. 8,21,29
Hemsley, J. 44
Henderson, J. 10,12
Henry, W.E. 8
Henwood, M. 5
Higgins, J. 38
Howe, D. 14,236
Hughes, B. 28
Hunt, A. 4,8,10,12
Hunter, D. 72
Jahoda, M. 49
Johnson, M. 41,78
Jolley, A. 26
Jones, K. 27
Judge, K. 24,35,39
Kay, N. 45
Kellaher, L. 32,41,42,68
Klein, R. 32,37
Knapp, M.R.J. 24,39,168
Laing, W. & Buisson, L. 34
Land, H. 8-10
Larder, D. 32
Leat, D. 35
Le Grand, J. 35,37
Leigh, A. 41
Leonard, P. 4
Lieberman, M. 27,28,110,133
Loney, M. 7,12
Lowther, C.P. 26
Mabon, G. 45
McKenzie, S. 51
MacLennan, W.J. 29
MacNicol, J. 3
MacPherson, I. 72
Marshall, T.H. 12
Maynard, A. 39
McCoy, P. 3,19,29,32,42,51
McKeganey, N.P. 72
Meacher, M. 21,40
Means, R. & Smith, R. 15-17,21,22
Midwinter, E. 37
Miller, E.J. & Gwynne, G.V. 21,26
Minford, P. 10,39
Mitchell, S. & Earwiker, J. 28-30
Moore, J. 37
Moroney, R.M. 5,6,9,12,121
Murray, N. 41

Neill, J. 26,29,30,212
Nissel, M. & Bonnerjea, L. 10,12
Norman, A. 27,89
Norton, A. 2,4

Ovenstone, I.M.K. & Bean, P.T.A. 26,177

Papadakis, E. & Taylor-Gooby, P. 7,32,35,36,39
Parker, R. 8-10
Parkes, C.M. 27
Parsloe, P. 14
Parsons, M. 43
Paterson, L. 29,30,177
Peace, S.M. 68,95

Peacock, A.T. & Wiseman, J. 6
Peaker, C. 35
Phillips, D. & Vincent, J. 36,38,39, 45,78,88,199,200,219
Phillipson, C. 2-5,13-15,17
Pinker, R. 39
Plank, D. 26
Pope, P. 27

Queshri, H. & Walker, A. 10

Reid, J.W. & Epstein, L. 15
Robb, B. 21
Robinson, R. 7,35,37
Room, G. 35
Rosser, C. & Harris, C. 8
Rossiter, C. & Wicks, M. 4,8,11
Rowlings, C. 17,25

Sainsbury, E. 16
Salvage, A. 8,13
Sawyer, L. 67
Sheldon, J.
Shanas, E. 4,22
Shaw, I. & Walton, R. 27
Sinclair, I. 5,21,29,149
Skipworth, G. 56
Stapleton, B. 30
Stevenson, O. & Parsloe, P. 14
Strauss, A. 62

Taft, J. 236
Taylor-Gooby, F. 7,32,35,36,39
Thatcher, M. 10,13,37,90,176
Thomson, D. 6,7
Tibbenham, A. & Phillips, D. 38
Tinker, A. 4,8,39
Titmuss, R. 3,7,36
Tobin, S. & Lieberman, M. 27,28, 110,133
Tong, M.S. 30
Townsend, P. 8,9,15,19-22,25,29, 98,99,133

Vickers, J. & Yarrow, G. 38
Vincent, J., Tibbenham, A. & Phillips, D. 38
Vladeck, B.C. 40
Wade, B., Sawyer, L. & Bell, J. 67, 101,133

Walker, A. 2,3,5,6,8-10,12,13,34-36, 38,39,85
Wall, R. 4
Walton, J.K. 27
Warburton 15,16
Ward, L. 25
Weale, A. 35
Weaver, T. 28,36-38,45,88,133
Webb, A. 35
Wedderburn, D. 8,22
Wilding, 7,29
Wenger, C.G. 8
West, P. 11,13
White, J. 56
Wicks, M. 4,5,8-11
Wilkin, D. & Jolley, D. 26,46,66
Willcocks, D. 5,8,20,25-29,45,59,68, 84,93,101,133,166,223
Williams, G. 78
Willmott, P. 8
Wiseman, J. 6
Whitney, R. 37
Wright, F. 9

Yarrow, G. 38
Young, M. & Willmott, P. 8

Subject index

abuse 35,40,42,43,106,126-128
admission
rates of 9
source of 137,150,151,202
stages 26,177-179
advertising 74,78,173,178,230
age 2-5,8,10,11,14,15,17,19,20,51,58,59,81,82,85,86,92,93,95,96,102,107,110,117,122,146,156,164,165,193,201,220,227,228
allocation system 60,163,172
applications 15,30
assessment
need 25,26,38,45,151,216,222,237,242
professional26,59,60,151,154,177,182,191,199,200,223,230,233,235,242
Audit Commission 5,23,24,32,240,242,244
autonomy 23,26,41,86,236

BASW 41,43-45,209,224,235
bereavement 14,27,71,96,122,131,132,134,153,155,197,221
Beveridge Report 9

Camden 40
casework 15,27,241
Central Council for Education and Training in Social Work 28
Centre for Environmental and Social Studies on Ageing 42
Chronically Sick and Disabled Persons Act 124
commodification 46
community care 3-5,9-13,16,22-24,32,38,42,119,146,147,149,151,152,154-156,158,172,173,216,218,224
Community Care Act 177,239,243,244
Community Psychiatric Nurse 65,127,207,214,219
consumers 8,23,35,37,38,43,46,153,170,172,174,192,220,222,228,230,232
cost-effectiveness 13,16,24,240,242
counselling 15,17,27,42,235,242

Crichton Royal Behavioural Rating Scale 66
Daily Telegraph 40

day care 23,36,57,119,127,135,163, 209
demography 8
Department of Health 51
Department of Health and Social Security 4,9-11,13,22-24, 32,34,35,39,41,43,45,46,70,85,98, 100,110,111,154,182-184,190,198, 211,220,222,224,225,228,229,232, 235,237
Devon 38,199
disability 4,8,15,16,51,180,195
disengagement 8,14,85
district nurse (D/N) 65,119,149
domiciliaryservices4,12,17,22,113, 143

Eastern Evening News 40
Economic and Social Research Council 48
economy 3,13,35,37,45,177,240, 242,243
efficiency 24,39,47,242
Equal Opportunities Commission (EOC) 11

Felixstowe 116,134
Firth Report 32,45,46,224,237
friends 5,11,116,118,120,125,131, 135,137,144,147,157,167,209,210
funding 7,32,34,35,98-100,110,111, 153,154,182-184,189,190,225,226, 228,232,234,243

gatekeeper 17,45,68,161,177,201, 203,206,213,216,222,231,232
gender 58,92,95-97,102,103,107, 146
General Practitioner 65,84,87,119, 154,177,181
Griffiths Report 9-11,13,222,225, 235,237
grounded theory 62,63
growing older 10,35,125
guardianship 106,136,163

happiness 3,59,68,73,169,170
Health Advisory Service 3
Her Majesty's Stationery Office 6
home help 12,17,22,24,65,103, 104,119,128,137,143,149,153-155,162
home life 40,41,70,73,170,188,195
home owner 34,36-38,41,45,50,60-62,64,68-70,72-74,76,78-90,92, 103,104,106,108-110,115,126, 128,131,140,144,154,165-168,172, 173,176-186,188-192,198,206,209-214,217,218,222-225,228-232,234, 237
Home Owners Association 41
home ownership 37,110,190,227
hospital care
costs 21
House of Commons 37,40

incontinence 4,21,67,87,101-104, 106,108,109,126,185,188
Independent Television 39,84
inspection 7,41,43,70,198,225
Ipswich 53,56,57,75,134

Kent Community Care Scheme 16, 22

Labour Party 37
loneliness 69,117,122,132,153,155, 166,221
loss 14,16,21,28,30,71,96,114,123-125,127,131,132,134,155,197

marital status 58,59,92,96,97,107, 146,201,227
meals on wheels 22,23,119,135,143, 149,154,155
medical ethos 88,188
mental deterioration 108,113,122, 123,125,129,130,134,135,139
Mental Health Act 134,136
mental state 58,67,92,104,106,108, 110,112,113,127,130,135,139,164, 165,180,185,191,209,227,232
mobility 4,21,67,101,102,114,116, 124,143,184,185,194

National Assistance Act 19,225
National Health Service 21,83,244

National Union of Public Employees 39,40,73,84
neighbours 11,103,118,119,128,131, 136,144,155,192,197
new right 7,12
Norfolk 36,42,49
Nuffield Foundation 20
nursing homes 34,90,133,147,172, 181,188,224

occupation 59,67,80,97,98,109
Occupational Therapist 65,124,143, 155,220
Office of Public Census Surveys 2,4,5,97
Officer-in-Charge 60,61,65,83,163, 241

pensions 4,19,37,110
physical condition, physical deterioration 67,92,101-104,123, 124,164
poor law 8,19,20
privacy 23,40,61,70,85-90,144,146, 160,168,174,182,184,199,229,232, 234,238
private residential home-function
 form 73,74
 location 75-78
privatization 5,7,32,34,35,37,60, 203,208,234,243
profit 13,39,40,46,82-84,88-90, 164,208,218
public expenditure 5,6,15,22,32,39
Public Health Act 134

Ratecapping 32
Registered Homes Act 40,41,43
registration 41,43,74,164,225
registration officers 41,47,61,70
Retirement Security Ltd. 78
risk 9,16,22,25,26,36,85,86,89, 117,129,136,143,195,199,207, 218,229,240
Royal Commission on the Population 3

S. Glamorgan 27,166,193,228,240
satisfaction 50,59,68,82,89,169,170, 229,238
security 7,87,118,146,168,173,199, 208,221,225,229
Seebohm Committee 22
self-determination 28,172,219,221, 222,242
social class 67,92,97-100,109-112, 140,189,222,227
Social Services Inspectorate 43
social work role 16-18,25,28,30,46, 69,191,222,239
social workers 1,13-18,22,25-31,43-47,50,58,60,65,69,70,103,117-119, 121,125-127,129,134-136,138,143, 149,151,152,154-156,158,161-164, 177,178,180,181,190-192,199-228, 230-233,235-238,239-244
Southwark 40
Stowmarket 75,76
supplementary benefits 7,32,34-36, 38,44,46,98,182,183,215

Trade Unions 22,73,83
The Guardian 37,84,90
The Times 44
The Way Forward 35

United States 78
University of East Anglia 48,61

vacancy 29,30,123,124,128,129,132, 136,140,143,156,159,161-163,165-168,173,180,197,198,206,209,211, 212,217,219-222,231,232,234
Victorian values 7
voluntary bodies 11
voluntary homes 44,53,116,237
volunteers 16,220

Wagner Committee 174
Wagner Report 24,32,222,237
waiting lists 156,157,161,179,180, 206,210,220
welfare pluralism 35,42
Wimpey 78
women 2,9,10,80,93,95-97,102,107, 109,110,117,120,127,131,140,144,